LOVE YOURSELF
& LOSE WEIGHT

LOVE YOURSELF & LOSE WEIGHT

The success story of self love

Katie Lips

Get a free book!

As a thank you for buying Love Yourself & Lose Weight, I'd like to offer you a free book.

Seven Days to Self Love

Seven Days to Self Love is my free, no-nonsense guide to kickstarting a self love journey. Want to know how to go from feeling lack in the self love department to feeling head over heels in love with yourself in just seven days?

Seven Days to Self Love is yours for free if you head over to: www.loveyourselfandloseweight.com/7days

Get your free copy now!

It would be great if we lived in a world in which we all loved ourselves and recognised just how awesome we are. It would be great if we lived in a world in which it was normal to talk openly and loudly about self love. We don't yet, so I've written this book to get you thinking about it, talking about it, and so head over heels in love with yourself that you can achieve anything.

With all the love in the world.

I'm so extremely grateful to the wonderful gang of people who've helped me write this book.

Thanks to my editor Lucy for your words of wisdom.

Thanks to Jo for being a true friend.

Thanks to my husband Paul who had utter faith in me, and for your encouragement - not just to write, but to change everything.

And finally, a world of thanks and gratitude to my daughter Lana for your extreme beauty and inspiration.

CONTENTS

Preface

Hello! And welcome.

Welcome to my story about how I learned to love myself, and how my newly acquired self-love acted as a catalyst for massive weight loss. If you have some weight you'd like to lose I hope this resonates with you. I hope you may even find my story funny too!

I've written this book to share my story in the hope that it inspires others, and just as importantly, I have defined a set of self-love and weight loss principles for you to take, adapt and build into your life so that you can make the necessary changes to help you move towards your individual weight loss goal. I have found something that is so incredibly powerful, and that worked so well for me that not sharing it would be a travesty. Divulging my very personal story has been challenging, and at times I might have overshared a little, but I really want to show you how easy it is to learn to love yourself – and to achieve the weight that you desire.

In the first part of Love Yourself and Lose Weight (LYALW), I will talk specifically about my story, and how I used self-love to lose 85 lb to reach a healthy weight – or 6st 1lb or 29 kg depending on the measurements you are most familiar with (for the purpose of this book, I will stick with pounds).

Traditional weight loss programmes want you to follow a set of rules, but this is not what I'm offering here. You'll need to keep an open mind, especially when I talk about loving yourself more. If this idea scares you witless right now, that's okay, but stay with me, and make sure you complete the activities later on in the book.

You can complete the activities as you go, or read the book, then do the activities afterwards. The Your Success Story section is your book, your story to write about yourself based on my guiding principles of self-love. Use this book as you see fit. Keep it to yourself or share it, and please keep me updated on your progress as I'd love to hear just how LYALW is working for you, so get in touch over at www.loveyourselfandloseweight.com

Thank you for choosing to read my book, and I wish you all the love in the world - as you embark on your very own self-love journey.

Best wishes,

Katie, August 2021.

LOVE YOURSELF & LOSE WEIGHT

Success Stories

It's powerful stuff, this thing they call love, and in this section, I am going to tell you just how powerful it really is - and how anything is possible, I'm living proof of that. You too can harness self-love to achieve whatever you want.

You're Amazing!

You are amazing. You are a wonderful, beautiful, resourceful, tenacious, talented specimen of a human being who can achieve whatever you set your mind to. You are so amazing that you utterly deserve anything and everything that you set your heart on.

1

Sound good? I truly hope so, but while it may sound good, it may not be how you feel about yourself right now. In fact, this is something I am pretty sure about, because if you were feeling great right now, you probably wouldn't be reading this book. You are here for a reason. You are here because you want to lose weight, and you may also be doubting yourself. Quite simply, you haven't yet learnt the secret of self-love.

For anyone who doesn't completely love themselves, the 'you're amazing' stuff can be horribly awkward, annoying even. If you're here at the start of this book I doubt you believe you're amazing, or that you are utterly wonderful, and I doubt you fully believe you can achieve anything you desire. My bet is that you ain't feeling it in the 'I can achieve anything' department, because you don't love yourself. Or rather, I should say you don't love yourself all that much, just yet.

But you can learn to love yourself. Yes, really, you can. And, if you stick with me, I will share my unorthodox, revolutionary weight loss method. As part of this method you will learn to love yourself. You will wake up every day so totally in love with you that you'll be able to achieve anything, even losing weight.

I'm Amazing!

Okay, Okay, it is still, and always will be very cringey stating my amazingness, especially as we don't know each other very well just yet. But I'm gonna go with it, as compared to the me of several years ago, the me who was six stones heavier, the me of misery, the me of inaction and regret, and the me of self-doubt who really didn't like herself very much, I am bloody amazing.

I am amazing not because I lost weight - and this is very important, so I'm going to turn up the volume here: I am amazing simply because I love myself; and I show myself love. To lose 85 pounds (yes, I lost 85 pounds), I needed to love myself. I simply had to love myself, it was the only way. In order to write a book, I needed to love myself. And to write a book about losing 85 pounds, I really needed to love myself. A lot.

A while ago I was faced with a choice: lose weight and feel happy with myself or don't lose weight, probably gain more weight and continue to be miserable. I had been faced with that choice every day for many years. And every day for many years I chose to remain miserable. I chose to continue to overeat, to gain weight, and to wallow in self-pity, all while pretending I was totally fine and okay with myself. I chose to do this because I didn't love myself enough to choose the other path, to make the seemingly tougher choice, to do anything about the situation I was in. I simply didn't care enough about me.

But now I do. And what started with a simple decision to love myself has enabled me to lose a massive amount of weight and to achieve other amazing transformations in my life.

Love is Amazing!

Love is transformative and fundamentally what this book is all about. I believe love is an amazing catalyst for dramatic and sustainable change. I will share my story as I hope you too can fall in love with yourself and, as a result, achieve what you desire and deserve.

While other weight loss books are all about abstinence, strict regimes and restricting certain foods, this book is just about love. It is so powerful. With love on your side, you'll be able to achieve amazing results that simply wouldn't be possible otherwise, regardless of how strict your diet is.

Love conquers all, so let's go get it!

MY STORY

So, who am I and why on earth would you listen to me about how to lose weight? These are of course the kind of questions you really should ask when you take weight loss advice from a complete stranger. After all, who wants to read another book about weight loss, written by someone who's never lost weight or who's never wanted or needed to? I know I don't!

Let me tell you here, a little about my struggle. I have wanted to lose weight. I have needed to lose weight. I have tried to lose weight. I have succeeded in losing weight and I have failed. I have tried eating less and I have tried exercising more. Finally, after many years of struggling with my weight, I learned how to lose weight in a different way. My method flies in the face of conventional wisdom which seems to stipulate that weight loss is all about focusing on diet and exercise. Well, for me, at least, conventional wisdom didn't work; it failed me as it has failed millions of other people all over the world.

The focus on diet and exercise entirely fails to even acknowledge that to lose weight you need to work first on changing your mindset. If you simply change your diet and start to exercise, you might well achieve some short-term success, but you haven't really got to the root of the problem. Your mind still thinks in the same way. This approach does nothing to address the issues that caused you to gain weight in the first place. This might sound harsh, but if you don't change your mindset, after a while, you will just go back to the way you were before.

I have been through the cycle of yo-yo dieting throughout my thirties. I am now 45, and as I write this am a healthy, and more importantly, a happy weight for me. At 5'6" my weight is under 154 pounds, under 11 stones and under a BMI of 25. I'm a UK size 12 and I am able to buy the clothes I like rather than the ones that will fit. I'm happy at this weight and while I still have some weight I could lose, I know that if I spent the rest of my life at this weight I'd have no regrets.

But it wasn't always this way for me. I used to wake up every morning full of regret; I'd get dressed each day full of regret, I'd shop reluctantly and hide behind layers of scarves, coats, big hair and bravado.

I had never been skinny as a child although I had never been fat either. As a student I lost weight and felt good in small clothes, but in my mid twenties I started putting on a few pounds. And it really was just a few pounds, nothing dramatic, I was probably still wearing medium clothes and no one would have thought I was big. At this time my social life was hectic, stressful and full-on. There was a lot of drinking, and a lot of eating to make up for the drinking and so the pounds continued to pile on. By the age of 30 I was struggling. I was wearing at least a size 16 and I was miserable in my own skin. I felt sad and upset with myself but outwardly I pretended I didn't care. I pretended I didn't want to look good in nice clothes, that it didn't matter and that I was fine.

I wasn't fine, I was the opposite of fine. I felt a sense of unfairness, I felt angry and all this negative feeling impacted me in other ways. I felt uncomfortable around my thin friends, I hated going anywhere where people dressed up or made an effort, I lost my interest in clothes and in looking good, and I struggled to achieve my professional ambitions as I let my low self esteem hold me back.

I worked hard to lose weight. I struggled. I lost weight. At one point I lost about 40 pounds only to put it back. I starved myself and went from a UK dress size 18 to 14-16 but the effort to required to keep going or maintain was too much and I put the weight back again and some. I was miserable when I was heavy, optimistic as I was shedding the pounds, and then miserable again when I put it all back on. I felt like an absolute failure, and I really didn't like myself very much.

Then everything changed. At my heaviest weight ever, of around 17 stones (238 lb), I suddenly discovered the art of long-term, successful weight loss. The secret was love. Instead of being so hard on myself, and mentally beating myself up, I decided to like myself. And my new-found self-regard eventually turned itself into self-love.

Over a period of 16 months, I slowly, patiently, and enjoyably lost over 85 pounds. I did this by learning more and more about self-love and I practised this idea day after day. That was over 6 years ago and while I have fluctuated a little in the years since, today I am most definitely at least 85 pounds lighter than I was when I started.

I'll be honest with you; it wasn't just a case of telling myself I was awesome or repeating affirmations over and over in the mirror each morning. I hadn't tricked myself into thinking I was amazing when I still weighed and looked the same. No, self-love is a catalyst, but it's not the end game. Self-love enables us to care enough about ourselves to do what it takes to achieve our goals.

It's also important to note that this journey towards self-love, and eventual weight loss, wasn't something that happened smoothly either or something that I achieved all at once. I didn't drop the 85 pounds and keep it all off for years afterwards. Nope, like so many of us, I did fluctuate - to the tune of about 20 pounds, then lost it again, then put it on again.

When I put a little weight on for a second time I thought long and hard about what had happened. I realised I was gaining weight because I had forgotten the most important thing I had learned when I initially lost all the weight. What led me to put a little weight back on was that I was in a toxic work situation at the time which jolted my confidence and made me miserable.

I was working really hard to save money and doing a difficult job that involved lots of commuting. Every day I would drag myself across London to get to work for a boss who insulted and upset everyone he encountered. The entire team suffered stress and fatigue, it was not even personal. The effects of being in a toxic situation with no time to decompress meant I forgot the key to staying healthy and happy. With someone telling me everyday that they didn't value the work I was doing, I stopped loving myself. I allowed other people's nonsense to dent my sense of self-love. So, I left that job, remembered to love myself, and hey presto, the weight was easy to lose.

I knew then that I had cracked it: I realised without an iota of doubt that for me weight loss starts with self-love. If I love myself, then I can lose weight easily and enjoyably because I want to treat myself right. I want to treat myself like the person I love most in the world.

It then started to dawn on me that what had worked so effectively for me could also help other people too. The questions kept buzzing in my head. Could I really help other people to lose weight? How would I do that? How would I share my story?? The first step was simply knowing that I wanted to help people like me all over the world to lose weight and to be happy. I decided to help others just like I decided to lose weight; I was clear in my intent, I made my decision, then I made it happen. I wrote this book to help people. I hope it can help you and I truly believe it will.

Love Yourself and Lose Weight is the story of my personal struggle and success with weight loss. It is guided by a set of principles that you can use if you are someone who wants to learn to love yourself, to lose weight, and to maintain a healthy, happy lifestyle.

YOUR STORY

You are reading a book about self-love and weight loss, so the chances are you're interested in one or both topics. I hope you're interested in both, in the same way that I hope you're open to considering new things and ideas that go against conventional weight loss wisdom. My challenge is to convince you to take the leap of faith and to believe me when I say that success in the weight loss game starts with self-love. I hope my story will resonate with you; perhaps we have some things in common?

Maybe you're sick of being overweight in the same way that I was. Perhaps, like I was, you're miserable about your weight but you pretend to yourself and to everyone around you that you're okay, although deep down, this is seriously affecting your quality of life. Perhaps, like I was, you're ready now for change. Perhaps you don't love yourself enough right now, perhaps you don't love yourself at all.

You can change that. You can learn to love yourself. You can learn to love yourself so that you start treating yourself with respect and loving yourself in the same way that you would the person you care about most in the world. Because self-love really can transform how you think about yourself. It can enable you to do things you never would have thought was possible. It can motivate you to try new things, to persevere, to succeed, and to enjoy the positive change.

The very fact that you are reading this means that you are at a crucial stage in your weight loss story. This is where you get to swoop in as the hero or heroine to figure out what needs to happen for the mission to succeed before hitting the home run. You have the power to shape this important story, and to make it a dazzling read. You have the power to make a dramatic change in your life.

However long you have struggled with your weight, and no matter how much weight you want to lose, or how you feel about yourself today, I want you to know that it is possible to stop the struggle, to lose the weight and to feel amazing. The way to do this is with self-love.

Often, when we are struggling with our weight, we simply add to the problem by telling ourselves a bunch of unhelpful stories. Stories like 'we're not worth it' or 'we don't deserve to be slim' or 'it's too hard for us'. These stories can stop us from making changes. We need to break free from these negative narratives that are undoubtedly holding us back. We need to replace them with much more empowering stories.

Whatever your story has been so far, this is your chance to change it, to write the next chapter just how you like. Instead of being the overweight person who was miserable but couldn't make a change, you can become the happy, healthy person who has a great life.

Yes, you can.

You can do all these things because you're amazing. You are an amazing, worthwhile person who deserves to be happy and to be whatever weight you desire.

Let's write your story here: I deserve to be the weight I desire, and I deserve to love myself. I deserve to feel freaking amazing!

The Weight Gain Problem

There are many reasons why someone puts on weight. We're all different, so your reasons may not be my reasons and vice versa. In this section, I will explore the reasons why we gain weight. It's not always just about food, either. The biggest problem, I find, is that as a society we seem to think the solution is simply eating less. We seem to imagine that this is easy and that people who have put weight on are a bit dumb. Well, guess what, it just isn't as simple as that.

We ain't stupid

We (anyone who's ever been overweight) are not stupid, yet so many of us are overweight.

In England, 28.7% of adults are obese[1]. A further 35.6% are overweight but not obese. That means 64.3% of us or almost two-thirds of British adults are either overweight or obese. In the USA 30.9% of adults are obese[2], with a further 35.0% overweight but not obese. That's a total of 65.9% the population who are either overweight or obese. Just in case you are not aware what is technically meant by obesity, it is a term that refers to anyone who has a body mass (weight) index (BMI) of over 30, and overweight is a BMI of between 25 and 29.9. According to British health experts, a healthy BMI is anything between 18.5 and 24.9. So, the statistics show that more than 60% of us are carrying more weight than is healthy – and I would vouch that most overweight people are miserable about that.

Obesity is an awful problem, and one that has so many terrible solutions attached to it. Most of these so-called 'solutions' focus on the mechanics of losing weight

---

1 https://commonslibrary.parliament.uk/research-briefings/sn03336/

2 https://nccd.cdc.gov

and totally neglect to examine why people become overweight in the first place. The mechanics of losing weight are known to us all, I hope. I mean, unless you've lived your life as a hermit, you're likely to understand that:

More calories in than you burn = weight gain
Fewer calories in than you burn = weight loss

Overweight people really aren't stupid, no matter what the media likes to suggest! No. We know we need to eat less and exercise more if we want to be lighter. Likewise, we understand that if we continue to eat more than we need, we will continue to get bigger. We also understand that if we were to eat fewer calories than we needed, we'd lose weight. Now, for anyone at this point who wants an 'all calories are not created equal' discussion, I will oblige you on this, but later in the book when I discuss the foods I eat to lose weight. You'll just have to keep reading to get to that bit.

Fundamentally, those of us who have gained weight know what being healthy looks like, what it means, and what it requires, but, for whatever reason, and maybe not even consciously, we have 'chosen' not to go down that path. No thank you! Not for us. Instead, us heavier people silently, begrudgingly, knowingly, resignedly, and sadly remain overweight.

For anyone who is screaming at this point, 'How dare you? I suffer from a serious medical condition that makes me put on weight even if I just eat lettuce', well yes, there are plenty of people like you out there. All sorts of people suffer from all sorts of diseases and conditions that mean they are more likely to put on weight and find it harder to lose weight. Often, people don't even know that they have such conditions and simply struggle on through. Yet whether you have a condition like hypothyroidism or polycystic ovary syndrome (PCOS), if you're overeating and not loving yourself, I hope I can help you fix those issues and be happier as a result. If you do suffer from a condition that makes it very difficult for you to lose weight, I believe self-love can help you learn to accept and work around your condition and make the changes necessary to achieve your goals. Most of us who put on weight though, do not suffer from a medical condition, other than, perhaps, a lack of self-love.

Telling someone who *knows* how to be healthy, how to be healthy is entirely pointless. We already know that if we lay off the carbs, and the pizza and ice cream, did some exercise, and limited our calorie intake, we would lose weight. But knowing is different from doing, isn't it?

Before I lost weight, my diet consisted of double portions of curry and rice, sneaking in chocolate bars when no one was looking and occasionally actually eating a salad just so I didn't look greedy. But it wasn't that I didn't *know* that this was what was causing me not to be a slender size 10. I really wasn't sitting there wondering why I couldn't buy any clothes in a regular store. It wasn't as if I was confused as to why I felt so bad about myself.

The doctors I saw over the years would go on about calories and exercise, but nothing they said ever made any difference to *why* I was overweight. It always seemed as if they just magically wanted me to weigh less so I'd be less of a burden on the health system. None of these conversations helped. In fact, any doctor who instigated 'the chat' only added to the problem - especially the thin ones who had clearly never gained weight or had any idea therefore why anyone else would. By reprimanding me about my size without remotely understanding why I might be overweight, they just made me feel misunderstood, isolated, and alone.

I certainly knew I was overweight, and I certainly understood the mechanics of weight loss (eating better food and moving more) but I certainly was not doing these things. So why not? Why was I, like so many millions of people, continuing to stay overweight??

THE REAL PROBLEM

For many people who struggle with their weight – what they are lacking is self-love rather than intelligence.

What I've learned is that when we become and then stay overweight it's because we're lacking love in our lives. I don't mean that nobody loves us, so we become fat. No. I mean that we aren't giving ourselves enough love. We just don't care for ourselves enough. We don't care enough to stay healthy, fit, and slim and we don't care enough to stop ourselves as we pile on the pounds. And we certainly don't love ourselves enough to turn that ship around, to reverse the damage and to lose weight. It takes a lot of positive energy to do any of those things.

We simply focus on the mechanics of losing weight because that's what we've been told we need to do. We were taught as kids that if we consume too many calories and don't burn them off, we will put on weight. I really do know that eating a calorie surplus makes me put on weight and that only a calorie deficit will make me lose it. Of course, it also helps if you get your calories from the right kinds of food - the type that makes you feel fuller for longer rather than the snacks that keep your blood sugar yo-yoing and convince you that you are hungry again 10 minutes later. Fundamentally, the art of weight loss is not rocket science: eat less food, do more and you will shift the weight. We know this!

The medical profession provides solutions that it knows technically will work, but it fails to understand why so many of us got here in the first place. In my experience, doctors don't understand, or more likely, they don't have the time to understand that there are reasons why we have put on weight, reasons why we have continued to put on weight and reasons why it's simply impossible to reverse that gain, and to start - never mind succeed in losing weight. These reasons are emotional, not physical. No amount of telling us about BMI, or calories, or that exercise might be fun, or that we're unhealthy is going to help until we fix the emotional issues that caused the weight gain in the first place.

When we put on weight, many of us enter the dangerous 'I don't care' territory. The 'I don't care enough about me mode'. It might start small, it might start by being triggered by an awful event, or a handful of minor disappointments, but it starts somewhere and then it spirals.

As we lose love for ourselves, we treat ourselves badly, we put on weight and the sense of 'don't care' is compounded - it just gets bigger. We care less and less. As we get bigger, we dislike ourselves even more until the very idea of self-love becomes alien, awkward, and something to shy away from.

When did I stop loving myself? When did I put on weight?

Self love and weight have been two battlegrounds in my life. And they are connected. In reality though, there's only one battleground and that's the self love battleground. A battleground? Yes, sadly it really has been, for me. While I have self love now, for large chunks of my life I really didn't have self love, self respect or high self esteem.

"Why not?" you may well ask, and many people do ask: "Why did you put on weight?", "What was the trigger?", "Did a bad thing happen?". It's not always easy to answer this. It's not ever easy to answer this, in all honesty.

I have written about this time and again to try to help myself understand what went 'wrong', what was missing or lacking, or what 'caused' weight gain. I've written about the fact that it was just a lack of self love that led me to gain weight gradually, that nothing majorly bad happened to me, that a few quite bad things happened near me and amounted to a dent in how I felt about myself, but none of the ways I was thinking about what happened, really explained what happened. Not to me, and not to you.

I think that if you're embarking on this journey with me I owe you more than that. I owe you more than a cursory glossing over of the issue, I owe you more, I owe myself more. So what did lead me to gain weight? What was my trigger, or terrible event that caused me to pile on the pounds? Having thought long and hard about this, through recent weeks, months and years I am now at the point where I can be honest with myself, and honest with you.

It started at the very early point at which I became self conscious. For me it was around age six. Like most of us at this age we start to notice difference - we start to notice how different we are from our friends. Some of them might be taller, skinnier, prettier, funnier, better at spelling, stronger, can run faster than us. Some of them might also be whinier, less approachable, less reliable, worse at Maths, and so on, but I noticed less where I was better than my friends, and was more concerned with where I was lacking. I developed a sense of being different at a young age.

When I was six, I was not any larger than the other kids: I had a different problem. I had eczema. This pretty common and less than exciting skin condition meant I had flaky knees, hands and eyes. I was an itchy scratchy child who was quite shy. I grew up knowing I wasn't massively pretty, I didn't have luscious flowing locks to plait and play with. I grew up wishing I didn't have the embarrassing eczema problem, wishing I didn't have to endlessly explain that it wasn't catching. At the tender age of six I couldn't understand that the situation would ever change, let alone having the emotional maturity to work on my own sense of self worth.

I was born in the seventies but did most of my growing up in the eighties. It was the era of the video recorder (we bet on Betamax) and of the microwave, of Pizza Hut versus Pizzaland, of an explosion of fast food, and of Lean Cuisine ready meals. We listened to Madonna, Jacko and Wham! and did aerobics, wearing shiny purple leotards. We drank diet drinks and used SunIn (a spray-in hair lightener) and crimpers without a care in the world.

At home, we were as healthy as the next family - well, not the ones who endlessly played tennis or whose parents played squash - no, they were definitely more into their fitness, but we knew not to eat too many of Grandma's Yorkshire puddings or helpings of apple pie. My sister and I grew up surrounded by family who took pride in their appearance, who strived to be slim.

Like so many kids, then just as ever, we learned fat was bad. We ate the Lean Cuisine ready meals. We believed it was important to be attractive and that attractive meant being thin.

In my teenage years, the eczema got better of course, and I grew up into a relatively attractive young woman, but I kept a sense of lack, a sense of being different from others, of not quite fitting in. I was still comparing myself, and in comparison to the ones with the long hair, the skinny ones who didn't feel the need to wrap a jumper around their waists to cover their behinds, the ones who exuded confidence, I felt different. Nowadays of course, we help kids at school to build their sense of self confidence, self worth, and I hope, self love, but back then it simply wasn't part of our education. Everyone just got on with it, I know this for sure, even my skinny friends felt inferior to someone or something at some point.

I spent a long time feeling unattractive and so I developed a coping mechanism. Instead of learning to understand that I was attractive just the way I was, instead of learning to love and accept myself, I developed the belief that it didn't matter how I felt about myself. I tried to reverse what I had learned growing up, and convinced myself that being attractive in a stereotypical way was undesirable. For many of us, looks don't matter, at least not so much as what's on the inside. We're all beautiful in our own way of course, but I managed to develop a belief that attractiveness wasn't desirable or applicable to me - simply as a defence mechanism.

Later, after I left school, I went to art college and university and something brilliant happened. I was surrounded by other non-traditional types and I fitted in. In this environment I learned to appreciate there were plenty of other people who were different too. My self esteem and confidence grew and I felt pretty good about myself. Coincidentally (or not) I lost weight and felt comfortable in my body - the most comfortable I've felt in my life until very recently. I was learning to like myself, comparing myself less to others, and accepting myself for who I was.

After university I entered the world of work. Like many of us, I had to shape-shift somewhat to fit into a new environment. I had switched the art college world for the tech world which, at the time was incredibly exciting. It was the early days of the internet. My early career was going well and I was confident and rather full of myself. Then I tried a new thing. Along with my now husband I launched a business. It was a huge deal for us and basically over a period of a few years, it failed. The business world I found myself in was less forgiving, and I was lost and lacking. I lacked business skills, money, the ability to present well to large audiences on big stages. The experience tested me so very much. I threw myself into it but kept getting knocked back. I felt knocked down and knocked out. I also felt very small in this big new world.

None of these things are that bad you might be screaming? 'Nothing awful happened to you!' You're right, I was lucky, I always found work when I needed it, I did interesting things, I travelled, I had people around me who loved me.

No, nothing awful happened to me. But around this time, there were negative, bad and absolutely awful things happening to people around me. Relatives and close friends died. I learned I wasn't immortal, or invincible. I learned life could be hard and cruel.

My sense of self worth was seriously low, and, out of resignation and rebellion, I found myself comfort eating. I was resigned to the fact that life was hard and I was rebelling. I'd comfort eat, and also I'd comfort drink. A lot of comfort. A lot of calories. A lot of weight gain.

I knew I was gaining weight and I continued to gain weight as I simply couldn't find the positive self love to lift me out of the malaise. I kept telling myself that it didn't matter that my business wasn't a success, that it didn't matter that I was gaining weight, that it didn't matter because it wasn't important to be attractive. I may even have convinced myself that being attractive was for dummies just to make gaining weight and feeling really unattractive ok somehow.

So while I grew up striving to be attractive, at some point, too many small (and some large things) tipped me over the edge, I felt I was losing or had lost the battle, and so I gave up and turned it all around in my tiny mind and got lost in a comfort eating mess. Now while being attractive is absolutely not the be all and end all, as someone who was perfectly attractive in reality, it was shocking that I opted to gain so much weight and basically give up on myself. I most definitely 'let myself go' and I most definitely sent everyone and the universe the message that I didn't love myself at all. And even though I was bloody miserable, without that self worth, self respect and self love I was unable to do anything to lose weight.

Without loving yourself, no amount of dietary knowledge or expertise, or basic maths for that matter, is going to help you lose weight. You have to love yourself to be able to say, 'enough!'. You need to love yourself just enough to make a start, to make a change. Loving yourself enough to read this book is a huge step. Reading a book about weight loss is an impressive first step on any weight loss journey.

The lack of love

A lack of self-love isn't always obvious to everyone else. In fact, you might come across as someone who is completely happy and appears to have their life sorted. But the problem might spill out in other ways, perhaps, as in my case, via angry outbursts, or just being constantly grumpy. And even if you do hold it together and are able to come across as calm and competent, your lack of self-love is something you can't ignore yourself.

As someone who has experienced a profound lack of self-love, I can share with you some of the kind of messages I was subconsciously telling myself:

- I don't ever think about how I love or care about myself.
- I don't really care about me.
- I'm not in control.
- I need to sort out this massive and awful problem, but I never get round to it.
- It doesn't matter.
- I don't matter.

My lack of self-love wasn't massively apparent to others until I got bigger. It was subtle and building, the fact that I didn't love myself led me to gain weight, the fact that I had gained weight further eroded my self-love.

Note that a lack of self-love is not self-hatred. I am not suggesting that anyone who doesn't love themselves feels hatred instead. No, it isn't that extreme. You don't need to hate yourself to treat yourself badly and put on weight. You just need to not love yourself enough. Without self-love you are completely ambivalent about yourself, and that's rather depressing. What an awful position to be in… not being excited to be you!

A lack of self-love stops you from enjoying yourself, from really loving being you, and being excited about what lies ahead. It stops you from welcoming joy into your life, grasping opportunities, and building relationships. And importantly, a lack of self-love can cause you to put on weight, and then to find it hard to lose again. Without self-love, it is hard for you to achieve the things you absolutely deserve.

Self-love is obvious to others. It's the thing that makes people attractive. Achieving self-love doesn't mean you have to suddenly become one of those braggy, arrogant types. You know the kind of person I mean: someone who struts about, busily telling everyone how wonderful they are when they probably don't love themselves that much at all. You really don't want to become one of them! To my mind, someone who genuinely loves themself is confident, friendly, polite, excited, positive, and dynamic, and the kind of person who brings out the best in others.

This is what self-love feels like:

- I think about myself in a positive light.
- I care about myself enough to treat myself well.
- I'm in control.
- I'm going to do something good for myself today.
- I want to do something good for someone else today.
- I'm working towards my goals, and I know I can achieve them.
- I've got this!

The link between self-love and weight loss is that self-love is the enabler, if you like. It enables you to lose weight as you're in control and you care enough about yourself to live well, to enjoy life and to achieve your goals. Fundamentally, gaining self-love shifts you from a position of not caring about yourself to caring enough about yourself so that you will do whatever it takes to give yourself the gift of weight loss, or anything else you desire, for that matter.

Self-love is effortless, and it's not mysterious or magical. In fact, with a little practice, it is something that everyone can acquire. I'm going to show you how to make a shift, to learn to love yourself and to lose weight easily.

MAKING CHOICES

If, as someone who is overweight, you aren't choosing to make a change, then are you actively deciding to stay overweight? Is that what you really want, and if so, why? Why are you not choosing to make the change? What kind of weirdo wouldn't choose to have a fit or even sexy body? What kind of masochist would choose to be fat?

I think it's fair to say that many people, especially slim people (and I don't mean to offend anyone here) who have never been overweight, just don't understand why others allow themselves to get big. But to be honest, I don't really think most overweight people get this either – in fact, they often see all those excess pounds as something that has just 'happened' to them rather than as something they have chosen. Often the weight just creeps up on you, doesn't it?

You were slim once. You were slim, then you put on just a few pounds. Then a year went by maybe, and you put on a handful more. Then another year went by. Then a decade flew by and not very suddenly, you're five stones overweight. It's not dramatic, it's a gradual process. In fact, it is slow enough for you to increase a size and be able to convince yourself that clothes are getting smaller without it being a big deal. That is until the dress is a size 18 or the top is an XXL – or a big number that you have always associated with fat people.

The fact is that overweight people don't consciously choose to be overweight, but by not doing anything to solve the problem, that is effectively what we're doing.

When I was overweight and heading towards morbid obesity, I never felt like it was my choice to be fat. I felt out of control, as if the weight gain was just happening to me, and I had no way of stopping it. It's not like I woke up every morning and said to myself: 'Hell, let's just get a bit bigger today.' It was more like it I woke up and ignored the issue because it was too big and scary to tackle. And believe me, I'd tell myself all sorts of crap to make it seem as if everything was okay – to convince myself that I wasn't choosing to be fat.

These are some of the total and utter lies I would tell myself:

- This is all okay, I'm not interested in being slim (this wasn't true.)
- I'm not actually that big (as I couldn't do up boots over my calves.)
- I look fine (I didn't.)
- I feel fine (I most definitely did not.)

- I don't care what other people think of me (it totally mattered to me that people would just see my size.)
- I really love food (I didn't actually love the food I was eating.)
- I could easily fix this if I wanted to (er… WTF!)

I was living in total denial. It wasn't that I was choosing to remain overweight, it was rather that I couldn't find it within me to make a choice to do anything about my weight problem. Every morning I woke up with regret that I was overweight, sad I'd have to feel uncomfortable in my clothes, but seemingly without the capacity to do anything about it. It was as if the problem was too big, too difficult, required too big a change that I simply couldn't face it.

I believe many people are in this same situation, the same limbo land of miserably sleepwalking towards getting bigger, and yet feeling completely unable to choose to change.

And it's a lack of self-love that is the culprit for this passive weight gain. This stops us from even being able to contemplate choice, let alone choosing to change. Until we learn how to love ourselves and start to feel some genuine self-love (which, by the way can come very quickly), it is impossible to even see that there is a choice to be made.

Well, the good news is that there is most definitely a choice, and once you start to love yourself, you'll be able to see it clearly. You will be able to make thousands of tiny positive choices with ease and achieve the weight loss you desire.

DIETS ALONE DON'T WORK

If I had once tried dieting and it had worked, I would not be writing this book right now. If it was easy to diet, to lose weight and keep it off, fewer people would be overweight, and living unhappily. If it was so easy to shed the pounds my Instagram followers wouldn't cheer me on every time I go for a slow, short run around the park or eat a tomato.

We know that diets don't work. We're over it. I am sick of hearing about the fact that diets don't work, especially whilst reading diet books. Diets are losing popularity and have been reinvented as communities or lifestyles. Authors of diet books are keen to establish their eating methods or way-of-life as 'not a diet', but they are really the same thing despite the re-branding.

I also believe diets don't work, at least not alone. It is true, however, that if you did manage to stick to a diet you would lose weight. If a diet restricts your calorie intake so much it creates a calorie deficit, then you would burn your stored fat to make up for it. You would lose weight. So why don't they work then, if, in theory their premise is so simple?

They don't work because they're often hard to stick to as they require you to eat foods that you are unused to, and to eat in new ways that don't fit your lifestyle. Or they specify that you eat foods that mean you lack energy and vibrancy, or they lock you into paying weekly to stay on track, or they make you crave the things you're not allowed to eat. They also fail because they focus purely on food, rather than on you.

They entirely fail to help you understand why you've put weight on in the first place, or to help you find the self-love you'll need to lose the weight.

To lose weight IS A BIG DEAL. Mechanically, it takes a calorie deficit, (eating fewer calories than you need) but to be able to lose weight, to keep it off and to achieve a healthy lifestyle for good, you need a bigger shift. Of course, you have to get the calorie deficit mechanic right, but you also need to have the right emotional environment.

My method focuses on those two key components - achieving the calorie deficit (the mechanics) AND creating the right emotional state. In fact, the emotional state must come first so that the calorie deficit bit becomes easy.

Right now, let's focus on diets, and why diets alone don't work, then we'll deal with how to create a positive emotional state that'll ensure you're capable of anything later. Before we can build the right emotional state, it's important to understand why a diet alone isn't going to help you and why you absolutely need more than they have to offer. My issues with diets are varied and numerous, but I've tried to keep it short and simple with regards to their shortcomings. It is important to say that some of these diets do work for some people, but for most of us we need something more. Below is a list of various diets, and why they don't work for me. I should know – I've tried them all!

Single Food Diets

Diets like the Cabbage Soup Diet, that only allow you to eat one or a few types of foods will leave you craving everything else. They might reduce your calorie intake for a few days, but in the long run, they are completely unsustainable. I might be able to eat cabbage soup for a couple of days (and I actually like cabbage) but no longer than that, surely!

Location Based Diets

Diets that follow the cuisine of other places like The Mediterranean Diet are ooh so appealing but completely unrealistic. I live in rainy, soggy England. It is literally pelting down as I write, and I know that the tomatoes we planted a few months ago never made it into anything resembling a Spanish tomato; suffice to say they never made it onto a plate. Adopting a Mediterranean diet, or another diet from a faraway land doesn't work because we don't necessarily have access to the right foods, and more importantly, our climate means we'll want different foods. What happens in winter when we need something warming but the diet says it's tomato salad again?

Shakes

Drinking your food in a shake or smoothie is not the same as eating. And it will make you feel as if you are seriously unwell because you can't eat normal meals like everyone else. Other than using the odd protein shake as a snack to help you build muscle whilst losing fat, I am not a fan of drinking my dinner.

Points Systems

Diets that use their own food classification system are likely to be horribly confusing and are more about constructing something you need pay for, than about giving you any real nutritional benefit. I tried one of these points based diets relatively recently. I know it works wonderfully for some, but personally, I found counting points was confusing and unsustainable. Slim people don't go around counting the points in food!

Sinful Diets

Diets that treat some foods as naughty have never worked for me either. I am not a fan of instilling the idea that some foods are bad, but that you can eat bad food anyway. Surely if it's that bad, you shouldn't eat it.

Or maybe it's not bad? To my mind, eating a chocolate bar is a silly thing to do if you want to lose weight because it will give you a rush of sugar, which, when it's subsided will simply have you craving more sugar. It is true that it is possible to lose weight through a calorie restricted diet that includes chocolate, chips and so on, but in my opinion it's harder to lose weight while eating those foods. Eating those foods makes you want more of them; it's addictive, whereas eating healthy food is not addictive, it's just nourishing. Oh, and by the way, I absolutely do eat chocolate occasionally, but I don't rate diets that use the fact that you can still eat junk as a selling point.

Other people's meal plans

Diets that give you meal plans expecting you will follow what other people have specified as a balanced diet each day are likely to fail because, well, eating is personal. We all know what we like and we all like different things. Sticking to what someone else tells you to eat sounds like being in prison. It's not sustainable; at some point you'll have to decide for yourself what to eat. What then?

Hard work diets

Diets that expect you to do all the work in the kitchen don't really work in real life. I like to cook, and I like to eat healthy, delicious food, but I don't want to have to follow elaborate recipes three times a day. We need losing weight to be as easy as it possibly can be. I once subscribed to a food & recipe box that sent me a food parcel to cook three times a week. Whilst I liked the cooking bit at first, I don't have 30 to 60 minutes spare every dinner time and so after the initial excitement wore off, I went back to my old ways of needing speedier eats.

Diet drinks

Many of my overweight friends drink copious amounts of diet drinks. I was totally addicted to a popular brand of diet cola, but I gave it up as part of my weight loss plan. I believe (although I have no scientific evidence to back this up) that the bubbles bloated me, making me feel full, then I'd feel hungry afterwards. If you are trying to lose weight, the best drink you can drink is water, plain and simple.

Diet Pills

I hate to admit it, but I've also tried these. I am really not proud of this, but I was looking for a quick fix, and I'm afraid there isn't one. Nope, sorry, taking pills just makes you feel bloated. And miserable. And a bit sick. And a bit silly.

Restrictive Diets

Restrictive diets make you want the thing that's restricted (the thing you can't have) so you'll crave it even more, become completely miserable, and probably fall off the diet quite quickly. Controversially, as I love the idea behind keto that fat is not bad but carbs are, I simply couldn't do it. I found keto so hard as it restricted practically all carbs and whilst I don't eat many carbs, I wanted and perhaps needed a few. For me, it was too restrictive, and the 'eat as much fat as you want' rule meant I ate way too many sausages and ended up putting on weight as I couldn't get into ketosis (fat burning).

It's likely I was doing something 'wrong', but after the initial dramatic water loss, which had me running to the loo every 30 minutes or so, I just felt lethargic and greasy. Any diet that makes you count your macros (I needed to eat less than 20g of carbs per day to get into ketosis) is pretty hard going in my opinion.

It is important however, to explore why these diets don't work; and it's different for different people. Some of it is circumstantial, like having time to prepare food, or having access to the right ingredients. What most of these diets have in common is that they restrict what you eat and restricting what you eat asks you to make a massive change to your life. Massive changes are hard to implement, out of the ordinary, and possibly out of your comfort zone. In addition to making a big change, they need you to do that out of the ordinary thing for a long period of time. This is unsustainable for most people.

Some of these diets ask you to not just eat different foods, but to count what you're eating, keeping track, and using a new-fangled points system that's at odds with how we live our lives. Sure, many of us enjoy tracking and can even cope with calorie counting, but if this becomes overly complicated it is easy to get lost and to give up.

Many diets don't work because they are too restrictive, too taxing, too unnatural, and not really focused on eating healthily, just on achieving weight loss, as a quick fix, for a fee. There's a lot more to dieting than weight loss though, by the way; what you eat can radically improve your mood and energy levels, your complexion and even your sex drive. Weight is only part of the picture.

A GOOD DIET

Now we've looked at what makes a diet bad, let's talk about what makes a good diet. There are some fundamental principles that make some weight loss approaches more effective. The Love Yourself & Lose Weight method is not about restricting certain foods (although some foods are way better for losing weight than others), but it is focused on how you eat, not necessarily on what you eat.

I will outline the basic tenets of the LYALW method:

Intuitive Eating

Like me, you were probably brought up to eat three times a day – breakfast, lunch, and dinner. It is a standard pattern that has evolved over the years and became established to fit around working patterns – and would have made complete sense during the Industrial Revolution when workers needed to eat big meals to sustain their energy. But how relevant is that to your life today? My guess would be, not much.

The Love Yourself and Lose Weight method is based on intuitive eating - whereby you eat when you're hungry, regardless of whether it neatly correlates with a mealtime. To lose weight and to maintain it, I eat five or six times per day, and I tend to have two breakfasts!

Some days it seems like I am always eating but eating whenever I feel hungry means I am always able to give my body just what it needs. I never overload it My experience of weight loss is that by spacing the same number of calories over more 'meals' I am keeping my body on an even keel; never too hungry and never too full. Various studies have been unable to draw a firm conclusion of the benefits of six meals versus three meals per day, but I think it's personal, so I would advise you to listen to your body and to eat as often as is right for you.

Eat when you're hungry

This sounds like a silly one, but many overweight people often fail to do this. By not eating when you are hungry, you are telling your body that when you do eat, it better store the energy as fat as you don't know when you'll be eating again. This is raw, animal instinct at work here. It's nature's way of trying to protect you. The best thing you can do is to train your body to use the energy it gets is to eat when you are hungry.

Have breakfast

I know lots of overweight people who don't have breakfast. When I was obese, I often skipped breakfast. Now I never do. Eating breakfast (at breakfast time) or shortly after waking, literally wakes up your metabolism. It tells your body to start processing the food, burning the energy, and to get going.

When you eat

Eating too much food late at night before bed means your body won't use up that energy and will instead store it as fat. A recent study that advocates front loading your day food-wise made newspaper headlines although it has been called into question by the NHS[3]. To me, this idea of eating more in the morning and lighter meals in the evening makes sense, certainly my own experience is that when I was eating no or light breakfasts and lunches then eating larger meals later plus snacks in the evening, I was much bigger.

Eating slowly

The speed at which you eat could be the difference between feeling satisfied after eating half of what's on your plate, and routinely wolfing the entire plate down as quickly as possible and asking for seconds. Eating slowly is an amazing weapon in our weight loss arsenal. If you did nothing else at all, eating slowly would help you to appreciate the food you eat, notice how much of it you're eating, feel the feeling of being full, and therefore help you to stop eating sooner, meaning you'll eat less food.

---

3 https://www.nhs.uk/news/food-and-diet/should-we-eat-breakfast-like-a-king-and-dinner-like-a-pauper/

Eating pretty

Making food, even simple food look good can have a huge impact on how you feel about eating it. Meals that are sloppily thrown onto the plate are a turn-off, whereas food that is beautifully presented will make you appreciate your meal more. We all respond to visual cues so make the effort to present your food beautifully so you can enjoy how it looks as well as how it tastes.

Eating with love

Eating and self-love can work in unison. Imagine if every time you ate you reminded yourself of how much you loved yourself, how worthwhile and beautiful you are, how you can lose weight and deserve to lose weight - imagine how quickly you'd improve how you feel about yourself. By remembering each time that you eat to love yourself, you're giving yourself the opportunity to practise self-love three, or five or six times a day, every day.

Moving your body

Diet and exercise work brilliantly together when losing weight. To exercise well you need the right fuel. Exercising can make you work up an appetite, so you can really enjoy and metabolise your food. Of course, exercising your butt off (literally) will undoubtedly help you to get into shape, but don't worry - this method does not require you to suddenly become a marathon runner or to swim the channel. The kind of exercise I advocate is gentle and enjoyable and at your own pace. It's all part of getting your body working for you, not against you.

Changing how you eat can produce some dramatic results. But before you can even contemplate making the changes listed above, you must love yourself enough first. You have to love yourself enough to want to start something new, to even imagine that change is an option. Self-love makes that possible, it makes pretty much anything possible.

ALL THE LIES

Sometimes it's good to be angry, and I'm angry about all the utter lies we're continually sold about weight loss. We are fed these myths daily which makes it not only harder to lose weight but means that some of us will never even embark on a weight loss journey because we believe that losing weight is simply too difficult.

We've been told a whole load of nonsense, frankly, by the billion-dollar food industry, so we should be forgiven for believing some of the rubbish we've been bombarded with over the past few decades. I know I've fallen for a lot the lies and I am sure you've believed some of them too. Let's forgive ourselves for that; after all, the food giants have all the wealth in the world with which to brainwash us. We are, in many ways, defenceless against this mighty machine. The lies are outrageous but because they're told over and over again, we believe them. Well, now it's time to think for ourselves and to question some of the stuff we've come to believe as fact.

Let's look at some of the lies we have been told. I bet you believe some of them, while knowing deep down that they're not true at all.

Lie 1: Healthy food, which is harder and more expensive to produce, does not taste as good as unhealthy food. You probably believe that you should like a certain food just because everyone else does. 'Everyone loves cake. You must love cake too.'

Lie 2: Unhealthy food, which is cheap to produce, tastes amazing. 'Pizza is to die for.' Well, it is but not in that way.

Lie 3: It's a treat to eat cheap food with little nutritional value. 'You deserve this decadent, indulgent, luxurious ice cream'. If you believe treating yourself well is to over-indulge on cheap sugar.

Lie 4: Some foods are so good you're addicted to them: 'Once you pop…'

Lie 5: Eating foods that contain fat will make you fat and low-fat foods are good for you.

Lie 6: There are quick fix diets and exercise regimes that will help you lose weight quickly.

Lie 7: It's easy, and perfectly possible for you to follow a diet and exercise-based weight loss regime and lose weight without first improving your mental state. So why are so many of us still struggling to do this?

Lie 8: It's hard to lose weight so what you need is a personal programme that tells you what to eat. It may be hard to lose weight but having someone telling you what to eat is more likely to make you miserable.

Lie 9: It's impossible to lose weight and keep it off.

Lie 10: Losing weight is simply down to diet and exercise.

Right, before we go on, I just want to examine Lie 9 and Lie 10 in a bit more detail. Firstly Lie 9: apparently, it's impossible to lose weight and keep it off – with research you read about everywhere suggesting that 95% of dieters regain everything they have lost within three years. Well it turns out this statistic should be treated with extreme scepticism. It turns out, this widely quoted statistic came from a study of 100 people in 1959. As The New York Times pointed out in 1999[4], we should treat this statistic very sceptically indeed.

I imagine that there is an unknown but rather depressing statistic about the rate of people who regain weight through restrictive dieting, but that it is the restrictive dieting that is the issue here. I lost weight and six years later, I am the same weight, give or take a

---

4 https://www.nytimes.com/1999/05/25/health/95-regain-lost-weight-or-do-they.html

few pounds. Yes, I had some minor wobbles, and yes, I've had to lose a little of the weight again but six years after losing 85 pounds, I have lost 85 pounds.

I believe it is possible to lose weight and keep it off AS LONG AS you don't lose weight through a restrictive diet alone. Weight loss requires consistent change, it is not a quick fix, and when you reach your target weight you can't simply stop what you were doing and return to a terrible way of treating yourself. By learning to love yourself, you are much more likely to the keep weight off - because if you love yourself, you're gonna be so excited about continuing to treat yourself well. By loving yourself, you will have dealt with the demons of self-sabotage, self-doubt, not feeling worthy and so on.

Now let's look at that false narrative (Lie 10) of weight loss being purely determined by diet and exercise. I will start by pointing out that both the diet and exercise industries are huge money-making machines. I guess what I am saying is that there is less money to be made from challenging how people think. But to me, the psychological part is the most important – by simply changing your mindset, you really can achieve anything.

The weight loss industry doesn't focus on self-love because it's harder to package, and harder to sell. If you previously believed that losing weight was just down to diet and exercise, I hope I am now managing to convince you that this simply isn't the case. Your mind has a huge impact on you achieving your target weight.

So, as you can see, we have all been continually fed a lot of misinformation, and to some extent we have believed it. And you might think that if you know you've been fed a pack of lies you can now stop believing them, and undo those years of brainwashing and everything will be okay, right? Wrong!

Just as we have accepted the many false messages we have received over the years from the food industry, we have also been convinced by many of the stories we have told ourselves. Let's be honest here – we do tell ourselves stories. And sometimes the stories we tell ourselves are a complete load of bull. Oh yes, they are! Some of them are out and out lies.

Here are some of the lies I have told myself – all of them echoed by unconscious messages I had absorbed from the food industry:

- I love chocolate.
- Burgers are delicious.
- It's okay that I am addicted to chocolate because everyone is - all women are. It's normal to buy multipacks of Dairy Milk or Snickers chocolate

bars, to hide them from my family, then eat them in secret, because that's what women do.

- I love food way too much to lose weight.

Then there are the lies I have told myself about exercise (I hated PE at school):

- I am not the right shape for running.
- I hate moving my body.
- I loathe all forms of exercise.

Next, there are the lies I told myself to make me feel less useless about failing to tackle my weight problem:

- Losing weight is hard.
- I need willpower and I don't have it.
- I would have to give up alcohol and my social life is too important to me.
- I'll never be thin.
- My body is naturally curvaceous.

And finally, there are the lies I told myself to pretend I was okay:

- I am healthy because I eat some healthy food.
- I'm not that big.
- I don't want to be thin.
- I don't care that I'm fat.
- I am fine.

Well, guess what? I was not fine. I was miserable. I binge drank to numb the pain of being fat, then binge ate to numb the pain of binge drinking. A lot of binging, a lot of bullshit, a lot of numbing, a lot of pain. And absolutely no self-love.

THE WEIGHT GAIN PROBLEM RECAP

So, I hope we have established in this chapter that people who put on weight aren't stupid, that we all understand the concept of calories in and calories out, and that of course it's possible to lose weight simply by eating less food.

I hope you have also understood that diets alone won't work as people put on weight for a reason. If the reason you've put on weight is because you found yourself lacking self-love, then this is something you need to acquire if you ever want to actively decide to lose weight and keep it off.

The Weight Loss Solution

There is a solution to being overweight; it is brilliantly simple, and it's called self-love. In this chapter I will discuss the truth about what it takes to lose large amounts of weight and what I mean by self-love. I will also share with you the story of how I stumbled across this amazing special power, and how building self-love comes from within - you already have everything you need.

Good news: there is a solution!

Hard truth: it takes courage, consistency, and time.

If you are still looking for a quick fix, you know, of the 'Lose 80 pounds in a month whilst eating 3000 calories as you sit on the sofa all day' variety, then you're in the wrong place. If you follow the Love Yourself and Lose Weight method, I can't promise you that the process will be swift, although you will start to feel better quickly. I can't promise it will always be easy, losing weight and changing your attitude towards food, exercise, and yourself, takes time and practice, but it will get easier as you build in positive healthy habits from day 1.

I can't promise you that it will all be enjoyable either, as there will certainly be times when you will doubt yourself, or when things will take longer than you'd like, but it will be overwhelmingly satisfying as you reach goal after goal - dropping pounds and inches, wearing clothes you never thought you'd wear, and feeling more confident and happier in yourself.

The weight-loss industry is full of people who peddle quick fixes. Those people don't have your long-term wellbeing at heart. They want to sell you a product, but they care less about whether their product really works for you. Many of them do have products that will work for you in the short-term, but because they aren't a holistic solution, they fail to account for the need for self-love so the diet or exercise regime can't really embed itself in your life. I am not trying to scare you off, rather, I want you to have your eyes open to the truth. Losing weight is not about changing one thing, it's about changing you; changing how you eat, move, and feel about yourself. Change takes time and commitment.

I know from my own experience that successfully losing weight requires several elements:

Self-love

This really means that you have to have your own best interests at heart. You can act as your own fairy godmother or super-hero and treat yourself as you'd treat the person you love most in the world.

Good food

If you want to lose weight, you need to eat good quality (not cheap to produce), wholesome, unprocessed food consciously and slowly. I don't mean we all need to go out and shop in high end supermarkets or live off caviar. No, what I mean by 'good' food is that the food has nutritional value. It is good for you - rather than being good for the giant companies that produce it by the bucket load.

Exercise

You need to move your body to get your metabolism going and to provide you with all those happy endorphins and a sense of achievement.

A Calorie Deficit

This should not come as a shock to you, but you need to eat fewer calories than you consume if you want to lose weight.

Good Habits

It is time to build positive new activities and behaviours into your routine.

Resilience

You need to keep going even if you've had a bad day and desperately want to indulge yourself.

THE WILLPOWER MYTH

Often, when I have tried to lose weight, I have convinced myself that I have enough willpower to see my diet through. But, if you want to shift the flab, willpower is not what you need. Sorry, I should correct myself here: you do need some willpower; willpower to remind yourself that you love yourself and that weight loss is not only possible, it is achievable and enjoyable. But if you're putting yourself on a restrictive diet, you will need stacks of the stuff as it will be such an awful experience. In fact, you will have to dig very deep just to stick to it for a couple of hours.

Willpower is a bad thing. You may not hear that often. It's another lie we've been told that people need willpower to lose weight.

If you believe the 'bad thing you are doing' is a good thing, then you will need willpower not to do it. This could be smoking, drinking, or binge-eating. You think it's great, so you need to have lots of willpower to not do the thing you want to do 20 times a day, or every Friday night, or as often as possible. It is possible to use willpower to not smoke, drink or eat very much, but not smoking, not drinking, and not eating very much will be unpleasant this way.

If you diet and lose weight through willpower all you've done is restrict your intake of food for a while. Yes, you will lose weight, but as soon as you decide you've lost enough and stop dieting, the weight comes back because the willpower goes. Of course, without willpower you just want to eat the stuff that made you gain weight in the first place.

My method, or rather, your method does not require willpower. It doesn't require willpower because once you love yourself you won't need willpower. You will want to eat well, eat consciously and slowly, and move your body. You'll want to do these things and you'll achieve your goals as they get more and more ambitious. When you reach your target weight - the weight you may well not yet believe is possible, you won't want to stop. You won't continue losing weight forever as that would be unhealthy, but you will want to keep treating yourself well for ever because you love yourself.

There is no 'diet' to stop just because you reached a goal. There is no going back to shovelling in the cakes, crisps and sweets, because you will love yourself and because you love yourself, you won't want to do that. If no willpower is required and self-love will ensure you enjoy treating yourself well, what's the catch? Is there even a catch? Well, no, there's no catch, but I want to be clear about the scale of the change you are about to make. Because achieving substantial weight loss is about achieving substantial change. Perhaps for you it is about making massive changes to your life. It is certainly not going to be achieved through quick fixes. It is about changing what and how you think about yourself, what and how you eat and what and how you think about exercise. The Love Yourself and Lose Weight method will be enjoyable, but it does take commitment.

Commitment comes in the form of thinking long and hard about you. It comes in the form of thinking about yourself and your goals every day. It comes in the form of knowing your 'whys' and repeating your affirmations each morning to get yourself set up for the day ahead. It comes in the form of reminding yourself you love you - every time you eat. It comes in the form of facing some hard truths and busting some myths. It comes in the form of knowing what you want, deciding to get it and then getting it, every day. It comes in the form of enjoying and celebrating your successes and moving forward each day happy in the knowledge that you are amazing.

WHAT IS SELF-LOVE?

We have talked about the fact that you need self-love to make sustained changes, but what exactly do we mean by this? Self-love is loving yourself like you love the person in the world you love most. It's waking up in the morning knowing you're going to have a kick ass day, and then ending that day feeling better, fitter, happier, more energised, or even thinner than when you woke up. It's respecting you enough to really start taking care of yourself. It is recognising that you have the power and the ability to make a change and then to set that change in motion. It's knowing that whoever you used to be does not matter. You're the you of today, and today's you can do anything. It is a feeling of deep empowerment and of being in control. It's no more lies, no more bad stories, and no more bullshit.

Self-love is not telling yourself that you're happy to be overweight if that's not the case. Some people may be happy to be overweight, but I wasn't one of them and I bet you're not either as you're reading this book. Self love is not pretending. It is not telling people it's all fine, when you just feel uncomfortable crammed into 'skinny' jeans that don't fit and you can't wait to get out of and covered up with layer upon layer of sack shaped clothing hiding behind a big scarf. I'm recalling my outfit of choice when I was not loving myself all that much, stomping around in slouchy boots which I'd bought because more structured boots with a zip didn't go round my calves!

Self-love is not stuffing your face with food that will make you fat and miserable. It is not getting drunk to obliterate it all and putting off dealing with your problems for another day. Oh no it isn't that! Those are the things you do when you don't like yourself very much, and I should know because I've done all these things. I have spent years overeating for comfort, although the comfort was short-lived and eventually led to abject misery. I've drowned those miserable sorrows in bottles of wine to forget I felt fat. And it worked; when I was drunk, I didn't care, I felt okay, confident even, able to take on the world. We all feel like that when we're drunk. It isn't real and it always leads to a hangover.

For me, years of overeating for comfort led to years of drinking to forget. Drinking to forget led to years of waking up with a hangover and a desperate need, not just for diet cola, but for CARBS. I craved carbs when I had a hangover, and I ate them in huge amounts to try to pacify my hangover. I ate a large bread-based breakfast, snacks, a carb filled lunch, often I'd eat out - a burger and fries. I'd often eat a curry with rice that I refused to share with anyone, plus a naan and papadums on a Sunday to curb the horrors I'd inflicted on myself on Saturday night. Food led to drink and drink led to food. And so on. Endlessly.

And all of it led to me being someone I didn't love. I didn't even like myself very much. Yep, that girl was struggling. I put up barriers, was unfriendly to others, felt I had no need to make new friends.

I digress not because I like remembering all that misery or reminding myself of the not fitting into non-plus-size clothes, the pretending I didn't care what people thought of me, the takeaways. I digress because to really understand self-love, it is important to understand the absence of self-love.

It is not true that without self-love you have self-hate. No, you can simply not love yourself, feeling complete indifference rather than hatred. Not caring much about yourself is quite insidious, and as I have said it might not be something others can see or that you recognise necessarily yourself. It results in just a little bit of lowered ambition, just a glass or two too much of wine, or just a pudding after an already heavy meal. Well, so what – who cares anyway? It is just a little bit of not caring enough to lose a few pounds, and then a little bit more pretending that this isn't an issue.

Here are some typical signs that you don't really care much about yourself:

- You don't put yourself first.
- You may well put yourself last.
- You don't see yourself as a priority.
- You don't do things for yourself.
- You don't feel like you have all that much to give to yourself.
- You don't feel in control.

For me, self-love is simply about loving yourself enough to give yourself the life you want and deserve. Whatever that life is. It's loving yourself enough to imagine a time in the future when you will be the weight you want to be, or as fit as you want to be, or as happy as you deserve to be. When you have self-love, you know that the world is full of possibilities, that you can shape those possibilities, that you are able to imagine, create and deliver anything you desire. Loving yourself manifests in so many positive ways. These are some of them:

- The ability to imagine a bright future.
- Knowing change is possible.
- Being in control.
- Feeling empowered.
- Doing things for you.
- Treating yourself as a priority.
- Knowing you have everything you need to give yourself the life you deserve.

Knowing you would do anything for yourself, just as you would do anything for the person you love most in the world is a powerful feeling. It is time to treat yourself to the same sort of love as the people you cherish in your life; this might be your partner, your mum and dad or your kid. Most of us know this feeling. Most of us would call it 'unconditional love'. It doesn't matter what nonsense our beloved ones get up to, we adore them anyway because they're the people we love most in the world.

Self-love is feeling about yourself how you feel about that person you love most in the world. You'd do things for you. You'd get out of bed and instead of regretting the past, you'd change the future for you. You'd do all the things you need to do in a day to lose weight - if that's what you desired.

To understand what self-love is, try and imagine that there are two versions of you. There's a giving you and a taking you. Or a you that works hard to achieve the things the other you desires. One of you needs to help the other one. One of you needs to say:

"Okay, I hear you. I hear you don't want to be overweight anymore. You don't want to wake up every day feeling regret about your size or your inability to do up boots with a zip, or your fear of swimwear. I get that you want to feel attractive and proud of your achievements. Well, I love you. I love you because you're a worthwhile, fabulous, energetic, creative (insert your own fabulous adjectives here) person and I want you to succeed in your ambition. Hell, I want you to be happy. I want you to have that gift of waking up in the morning and instead of feeling regret, feeling a sense of calm. I want you to wake up every morning with a smile on your face, leap out of bed and throw on some clothes and look and feel great in them.

I am going to do whatever it takes simply because I love you. I have always loved you; I love you as you are today right now, I will love you tomorrow and the next day and the day after that. I love you enough to be creative about it, tenacious, hardworking, and passionate about giving you what you want. I want you to look back on today as the day I decided to do great things for you. Because I have decided, I am going to do whatever it takes. You want to be a healthy weight? Well, you can be a healthy weight, and what's more, you deserve to be the weight you want to be, and I love you so bloody much I'm gonna make sure you achieve your dreams. I'm gonna do whatever is in my power to make you happy."

See, this is powerful stuff. It's like having a guardian angel or a fairy godmother. The fabulous, achieving, giving version of you is going to make everything happen for you, creatively finding the resources and energy to do what it takes to make sure that the princess (or prince) will go to the ball.

SELF-LOVE VERSUS BODY POSITIVITY

I want to take a moment to explain the difference between self-love and body positivity. Body positivity is a great thing, but it really does just focus on your body, whereas self-love is all about you, regardless of your physical form. You could have a traditionally fit, slim body or be officially obese and either have self-love or not. Some people who are slim love themselves, some don't. Some people who are overweight love themselves, and again, some don't.

Body positivity is simply about your body, it's not about you as a person. It means loving your body whatever size or shape it is.

Self-love is about you regardless of your body - almost as if you were detached from it. Self-love is something that develops, based on a whole host of inputs and activities and it is about way more than just your body. It is about how amazing you are as a person. I salute anyone who finds self-love, including people who are overweight and who love their overweight bodies. I salute them because they have found self-love.

I dislike the argument that anyone who wants to lose weight or who helps others to lose weight is in some way fat shaming. There are many millions of people who are overweight and who are unhappy being overweight, and those people need help. I want to help them, and I dislike the idea that they are too afraid to say, 'I don't like being fat and I'm going to do something about it.'

I bet that most people who are overweight wish they were not, and while we should appreciate our bodies for the marvellous things they are, whatever their size, we shouldn't feel scared or embarrassed to say, 'I want to be smaller', or 'I want to be healthier'. For those of you who would prefer to lose weight, self love can help you achieve that - whereas body positivity can't.

THIS REALLY WORKS

Self-love helped me lose 85 pounds. And if it worked for me – it can work for you too.

When I got on the scales and saw that my weight had dropped to 10 st 13 lb, I felt such incredible joy, excitement, and relief. I had done it. I was no longer a government statistic, I was no longer obese, and I was no longer overweight, - I was finally, and for the first time in over a decade, a healthy weight. Admittedly, I was at the top of the healthy weight range with a BMI of 24.9, but at 5'6" and 10 st 13 lb I had reached my healthy weight goal.

Four weeks after I gave birth to my daughter in June 2014, I weighed 17 stones, and no this wasn't just 'baby weight', as I was already obese before I got pregnant, weighing around 15 stones, which was far too heavy for my medium 5ft 6ins frame. But I used my pregnancy as the perfect excuse to overeat – the hormones made me do it, of course they did! I remember stopping off at McDonalds for a large Quarter Pounder® with Cheese Meal before dinner most days. I felt compelled to eat bucket loads of fast food, and yet still believed that once my baby was born, I would somehow stop eating so much and miraculously become slim. I was in denial – and I was putting on a massive amount of weight.

As time went on, conversations with my midwife turned to my birth plan. The 'plan' was that I'd go to the big hospital 20 miles away as they had all the right facilities there to ensure an 'easy birth'. As a first (and last!) time mum, I wanted a hippy dippy natural birth in water, with soothing mood music. The midwife explained to me that I couldn't give birth in a birthing pool because I was too heavy to lift out if anything went wrong.

WHAAAAT? I was too heavy to lift out. Wow!!

I felt so angry that the National Health Service was going to ruin my birthing experience that I went home determined to look up the weight restrictions of birthing pools, with every intention of making a fuss. I never got round to it in the end. And, of course, all my ideals went out of the window once I went into labour. By that stage, I really was happy to go and get proper care and proper drugs at the big hospital with all its epidurals and the like. Mood music was nowhere to be heard.

It wasn't until after I had my daughter though, that my weight gain became fully apparent. The fact that she was all tucked up in her Moses basket as I stared at her lovingly meant she was no longer inside of me. So, the massive protrusion in front was not a baby after all, it was just fat. After the first few weeks of sleep deprivation, I looked in the mirror and instead of being confronted by a massive pregnant woman, there was just a massive fatty staring back at me. I was still wearing my maternity clothes because they were the only things I had that would fit.

When my daughter was a month old, my husband and I decided to go to out for a walk, lunch, and a spot of shopping, which felt like an epic adventure at the time. I went into a shop and bought a pair of jeans. I didn't try them on, as trying things on was often a hideous experience. I just bought them, hoping that the shop assistant wouldn't judge me. I bought size 18 (the largest in the shop) knowing they were extremely unlikely to fit. At home, I attempted, unsuccessfully to pour myself into them. I looked at the jeans. I looked at the baby. I looked at the jeans. I cried.

I was a UK size 20 (or perhaps larger), and I was utterly exhausted. But as I looked at my little girl and felt so much love for her, that crippling love that parents have, I realised that love could help me. It could help me get into those jeans.

Then I made a decision: 'I'm going to get into those jeans. I'm going to do it for you and I'm going to do it for me.' I said to her.

At that moment I felt overwhelmed with emotion, (most likely from the sleep deprivation), but I knew I needed to be there for her and to do that I needed to be there for me. I knew that being that big wasn't healthy for me, it was likely to shorten my life expectancy and was likely to limit my enjoyment; I'd be a fat mum. I didn't want her to have a fat mum. She deserved a slim mum; a mum who could take her swimming, a mum she wasn't ashamed of as she grew up, a mum who could run away from tigers. The love I had for my daughter enabled me to make a decision; it gave me the motivation to make lots of important changes to my life, and ultimately, to lose weight. I got into those size 18 jeans a few weeks later, having lost 20 lb.

As the months passed, I started to feel a sense of pride and achievement. I had worked hard to get into that pair of size 18 jeans, and I thoroughly enjoyed and savoured that moment of putting them on. It was great. What was next though? The size 18 jeans were still, after all, size 18 jeans, not exactly everyone's goal size. So why not size 16 jeans? Acting on impulse and instinct, I quickly ordered the same jeans in a size 16, knowing it would be a while before I'd wear them, but wear them I would!

I had started my weight loss journey, and I was learning to love myself, but my confidence was still shaky, so I didn't confide in anyone what I was trying to do.

It takes focus

In the coming weeks, I was alone all day in the house with a baby who needed lots of attention, but there were times when she slept when I could focus on me and on losing weight. I thought carefully about what worked and what didn't work for me, and I devised a plan around food and eating. I started walking more and I started tracking my progress, creating a new goal each time I achieved one.

I ate good whole foods, and cut out all the processed junk, and I ate slowly and consciously which helped me to basically eat far less food. I started to move more too, doing more tidying, washing, and pottering around the house. But these were just the mechanics of weight loss (fewer calories in + exercise = weight loss) and whilst the mechanics worked, it was the love that I felt for my daughter that meant I could do this.

And at first, the love I felt was just for my baby. I didn't even think about loving myself. But as the size 16 jeans went on and I looked in the mirror I took a good long look at myself. I was a different person now, a mother, one that knew how to change a nappy and erect a pram in a couple of seconds with one hand. I was getting more confident, feeling capable and in control, and I liked what I saw. I liked myself. I was kind of cool.

In the next few months, I made every day, and every meal and every food choice count (eating delicious healthy food). I learned how to run again and kept losing weight. I was able to do this because of the growing love I had for myself. I started to talk to myself each morning - reminding myself of why I wanted and needed to lose weight, or why and how my life would be different when I was a healthy weight. This included telling myself nice things. Over time I became able to say, 'I love me' and over time I even believed it. I bought the size 14 jeans, then I bought the size 12 pair.

As I got on the scales 17 months after my daughter was born and finally crossed the line and became a healthy weight with a BMI of just under 25, I had learned to love myself. I'd lost 85 pounds and spent a lot of money on the same pair of jeans in four different sizes.

IT COMES FROM WITHIN

How much other people do or don't love you is irrelevant. Many of us value ourselves based on how much we think others value us. We link what others think of us to how we should think about ourselves. Plenty of chick flicks show girls unlucky in love, doubting their self-worth and reaching for the ice cream.

In our society, our ability to find a partner can determine our self-worth. We value love from others above all else. It is what keeps humanity going, after all, so we're naturally predisposed to value romantic love highly. We're taught from a young age that love conquers all, that we should strive to find a partner. We're taught that we should receive love from others and give love to others. But what I find utterly shocking is that we are not taught to love ourselves. How can we love others properly if we don't love ourselves?

Many of us can feel love from others and feel love for others yet we don't feel love for ourselves. It is also true that some people don't get much love from others, and yet, they can feel great love for themselves. Whilst it's true that loving yourself helps you attract love from - and give love to others, there should be no correlation between how much love you feel from others and how much love you feel for yourself.

You can love yourself even if no one else in the world loves you. Imagine that. Imagine sitting on your desert island all alone. You could be the kind of desert island dweller who sits miserably awaiting rescue, or you could be the kind of desert island dweller who decides to make the best of it, and creates a new home, building resources to rescue yourself. Even when there are no other people around, we need to love ourselves if we want to achieve our full potential.

A lack of love from others is no reason not to love yourself. In fact, a lack of love from others could be the perfect catalyst to love yourself even more.

Often, we rely on others too much to achieve things for ourselves anyway, and to give us validation. When we start a relationship, we expect the other person in our lives to be perfect and if they're not, we feel short changed. We're all imperfect, but it is what we do with our imperfections that makes us interesting and attractive, and what our bonkers, crazy personalities lead us to do with our lives that makes us loveable.

There will be times when the people we like or love, don't feel the same way about us. It is immensely tough but the worst thing we can do when this happens is to leap to the conclusion that there's something wrong with us, that we're to blame, that we're not loveable. There are millions of reasons the stars don't always align, and it's vital we build our own sense of self love to ensure we can give ourselves what we deserve in life.

No one is perfect. No one is going to appear like a knight in shining armour. Those things don't happen in real life. We don't live in a fairy tale. Except, that is, when we write our own; when we become our own knight in shining armour, or fairy godmother, when we wave our own magic wands, and cast our own spells - then we can indeed make our dreams come true.

Take responsibility for loving yourself!

Self-love is challenging in the sense that you are in control. There are no excuses, and there's nowhere to hide. You are responsible, you are accountable. Only you. No one else. You can't blame someone else for not loving you, you must take responsibility.

Think of the person you love most. What would you do for them? At this point we get all gushy and think of the lengths we'd go to for someone precious in our lives. I know I'd do absolutely anything for my daughter, which really did make giving up binge eating junk food a very small sacrifice indeed.

But would you do any of these things for yourself? Any of them? And if not, why not?

What would you give your favourite person for their birthday? Would you work hard to achieve something for them? Would you make a big change if they were in trouble? If they were overweight and needed to lose a lot of weight to improve their health and happiness, would you help them? What would you do to help them? How far would you go?

The odds are, you'd do big scary stuff for your favourite person. Well now it's time to make you your favourite person - and to do big scary stuff for you. Instead of feeling like this is a challenge too far, this should be empowering. You are capable of this. You can do it. With the power of self-love, you can achieve anything. You can certainly lose weight.

THE WEIGHT GAIN SOLUTION RECAP

Once you have moved away from the idea that weight is only about food or calories, you will begin to open your eyes to the fact that how you think about yourself has a lot to do with how you treat yourself. The fact is that the way you treat yourself will have a massive impact on your weight as well as your general wellbeing. It might seem obvious when you think about it, but so many people simply don't realise the importance of self-love.

I hope my story explains the principles of self-love in practice and I hope it resonates with you. But my story is just my story, yours will be different. You don't need to have a massive amount of weight to lose, you don't need to have children, or be a new mum to feel the love. You do need to recognise though, that self-love comes from within you, and that you certainly have the power to love yourself and to transform your life.

ACTIVITY

Now you're ready to get started, turn to Your Success Story. Fill in the details of your story as you know them so far. Do this, and you're on your journey. Congratulations!

Creating the Right Mindset

Now we get to the good bit, the part where you get the tools you need to learn to love yourself. As you build skills in self-love, you'll dramatically change how you feel about yourself. Anything will become possible. This section is a guide for getting ready to start loving yourself, and it covers your whys, creating effective affirmations and defining your goals.

There are activities to help you do these things in Your Success Story (Part 2 of the book). You can refer to the activities as you go or do them after reading the theory.

Up to you.

UNDERSTAND YOUR WHYS

Why do you want to lose weight?
Why do you want to lose weight really??

That sounds like a totally silly question. And your answers might be quite varied, such as 'I'd like to look great in a bikini', or 'I'd like to live to see 50', or 'I'd like to fit into an aeroplane seat'. While these may all seem like valid reasons on the surface, these are all rather superficial responses, and I'd like you to delve a little deeper.

You need to define your whys, as they are your guide; they will help you to know why you're doing what you need to do each day. Without a clearly defined why, you will just be flailing around, thinking weight loss might be a good idea, but not really having any clear reasons for going ahead.

If someone else has told you to lose weight, it's likely that other person has a why in mind for you, but unless it's also your why, any attempts at weight loss will be futile. They simply won't work as you won't be signed up to the mission.

As you embark on and continue with your weight loss journey you need to know, and truly know why you're doing this. Of course, having the body of a 20-year-old supermodel would be amazing, but that really is an unrealistic goal for most of us. Being healthy is important to most people, but why is it a priority for you?

When I was 85 pounds overweight, I wanted to lose weight so that I could fit into some size 18 jeans and feel less embarrassed about my size. I also wanted to be the best mother I could to my daughter. But these were goals rather than my specific whys. There was more to it than just those things for me, and there will be more to it for you too.

In order to really know your whys, you need to go deeper. Indulge me…

Why did I want to fit into these jeans? Because I didn't want to be someone who couldn't fit into clothes from a normal shop, and I really hated feeling like such a failure. I hated feeling ashamed. I hated feeling embarrassed.

Why did I want to be less embarrassed about my size?

Because having strangers stare at me because of my weight made me feel really self-conscious. And I wanted to be able to walk down the street without feeling like I needed a sit down – no, really, it's effortful lugging all that fat around!

Why did I want to be there for my child?

Because I'm a parent. And because I know that at some point, I'll have to go to a beach with the kid and wear a swimsuit and I don't want people feeling sorry for my child for having a fat mum. And I don't want to die before the kid is at least 40. And I don't want the kid to be fat. And I feel hopeless as a parent, and I don't want to fail this person who I love more than anything in the world.

Okay, now we're getting somewhere. Do you see where I'm coming from with this? It's important to go beyond the initial headline, to know what's really driving you. But, what a load of don't wants. What a load of misery!

Early, fledgling, first attempt whys often focus on what we don't want. We don't want the misery of being overweight. We don't want to go on wearing outsize clothes, we don't want to die prematurely, from a heart attack, eating a donut whilst doing the grocery shopping.

Look at the Positives

But what if we could shift from thinking and talking about the misery of being overweight to thinking and talking about a better, more positive kind of why? It's important to frame our whys as positives rather than just the lack of a negative. A lack of a negative just gets you back to zero, nothingness. Nada. Whereas by defining the positive things that are going to happen as you lose weight, you'll be much more driven; you'll have something good to aim for.

I honestly believe that an undefined why, or even a poorly defined one can scupper your chances of weight loss. If your why is just about removing something bad, such as the desire to feel less self-conscious, the end result isn't going to leave you feeling elated, or fantastic, or confident, or ecstatic. No, it just leaves you a little less self-conscious.

Unfortunately, if you have been feeling self conscious for years, decades even, you're used to feeling this way. You might feel self-conscious about not fitting in your clothes, or worried that people will judge you, or that you will judge yourself, and you will then feel miserable. But the truth is that if you are totally used to feeling self-conscious, worried, and miserable – these are all quite normal feelings for you. And although unpleasant, you can pretty much handle these feelings.

Well, you have had to, haven't you? This is a bit of a problem, because if your whys are all focused on removing negative feelings that you are pretty much comfortable with, you are kind of sending yourself mixed messages. You are telling yourself that whilst you'd like to remove these negative feelings, you don't really have to, as you can already live with them.

So, let's come up with some much more inspiring whys! How about starting with an awesome feeling or an amazing thing that you never dreamt could happen. How about that?

Why do you want to lose weight? My whys have changed over time but there are some common threads. My whys go a little like this:

I want to feel fabulous in my size 12 jeans and to revel in the knowledge that I can shop anywhere, even 'skinny girl shops' that are probably more appropriate for teenagers.

I want to feel confident in my body and proud of my appearance, as I catch sight of my reflection when I'm out and about. I want to be noticed by other people for looking good. Hell, I want to be lusted over! Why not? Seriously, why not?

I want to enjoy every moment with my daughter and to give her the childhood she deserves. I want to set a good example to her so she can grow up to love herself, to live well, and to be happy. I want to go to bed each night happy that she's happy. I want to enjoy and look forward to days by the beach or the pool.

ACTIVITY

Now you've learned about creating your whys, go to Activity 1 to define yours.

Saying Stuff Out Loud

Splurgh, yuck, sick. I know, talking about loving yourself is totally full of the awkwards.

As a society, we never talk about loving ourselves, do we?

We talk endlessly about loving other people, and we spend a disproportionate amount of our time trying to find people to love us, but we never talk about loving ourselves. It's as if we think loving ourselves is arrogant or offensive somehow. Our society seems to think people who value themselves a bit too much are immodest or self-obsessed. Really? It's as if we really ought NOT to love ourselves - as to do so would break some sort of sick social code whereby we all need to live miserably, thinking we're rubbish.

How and why do we feel like this? Why is loving ourselves not the thing we should all be doing? Why should we feel it's odd to love ourselves?? Honestly, I have no idea. And frankly it's ridiculous. We should celebrate ourselves; we should love ourselves, AND we should celebrate self-love. Here are some interesting facts on self-love:

- For some people, self-love comes easily.
- There are lots of people who do love themselves.
- Self-love doesn't come naturally to everyone.
- It's hard to achieve great things, or much at all, if you don't love yourself.
- Loving yourself is not at the expense of loving others.
- If you love yourself, you will likely love others more and receive more love from other people because you'll be emitting good vibes.

If you aren't a fully signed up member of the 'I know why self-love matters' club it's likely you're not head over heels in love with yourself. So, for anyone who doesn't love themselves 100%, here's how to start. To start feeling self-love, you can start small, find just a tiny seed of self-like, and build on it. Self-love can start with acknowledging you're a decent human, deserving of good things, and enjoying life.

POSITIVE AFFIRMATIONS

Ah yes, affirmations. Another icky awkward load of nonsense, yes? Not so. An affirmation is simply something you say to remind yourself of something important, and by repeating this message, you actually begin to live by it. Over time, if you say it often enough, you will believe it. You will realise how it helps you to get your head straight, helping you to remember why you're on this weight loss journey.

After a while, these affirmations will no longer seem naff, and you will look forward to saying them. Honestly, however silly they might sound in the beginning, affirmations really do work because if you repeat them often enough, our brains begin to accept their messages as facts. Once your brain knows that you are worthwhile, and deserving of a fabulous healthy body, and need to fit into your skinny jeans, your brain obliges and will help you get there. Don't just take my word for it, there is plenty of evidence[5] that suggests affirmations work.

---

5 https://positivepsychology.com/daily-affirmations/

ACTIVITY

Activity 2 will help you define your affirmation in just a few easy steps.

Now, once you've defined it, say your affirmation out loud. Go on, it won't be that bad! If you are simply laughing your arse off right now, that's okay; I was not your typical affirmation sort of a girl when I started this journey. I thought people who repeated positive thoughts to themselves in the mirror were bonkers if I'm honest. But I was wrong. And it's okay to be wrong and to change your mind.

When I started to address the fact that I was lacking in the self- love department, I knew that starting by telling myself I loved myself was a great first step, so I tried it. At first, it felt a little uncomfortable. Not dishonest, but certainly a little awkward. I felt uneasy. But over time I practised, and practice made it feel less icky. I developed a simple couple of sentences that I repeated to myself every day. Initially, I felt a little embarrassed about it, but after a week or so, it felt okay. And after a couple of weeks, guess what? I started to believe what I was telling myself. As the weeks passed and as the effects of loving myself were plain for everyone to see, I really began to believe the messages I was telling myself. That is the power of self-love.

Here I will share with you a couple of my regular affirmations, just so you can see how simple they can be:

I love me.
I am awesome.
I deserve to have a slim, healthy body and to feel great about it.

ACTIVITY

Even if you're completely terrified of saying your affirmation out loud, give it a go. Activity 3 will help you to get chatty with yourself.

THE DECISION TO LOVE YOURSELF & LOSE WEIGHT

When you decide to love yourself and lose weight you'll never need to look back. Sounds good, doesn't it? Well, it really is. The act of deciding to love yourself means you will love yourself, the act of deciding to lose weight means you will lose weight; the weight will just automatically, magically, go.

A decision is powerful. A decision is a commitment. A decision tells your brain, and the universe for that matter, what is going to happen.

If you're thinking this sounds too good to be true, it could be because you don't yet fully understand the utter power of a decision. A decision is different from a desire, or longing, or a vague ambition; a decision is an absolute commitment, and a commitment means that whatever you decide will get done.

Unless you really decide to do something, anything, you aren't really committed to doing it. If you haven't decided to do something, you haven't told your brain what to do. You're still just thinking about it. Just thinking about losing weight and wanting to lose weight but not actually committing to the fact that this is absolutely what is going to happen, won't be enough for you to achieve your weight loss goals.

Now, you may imagine that all this thinking about something would mean that change happens, but this is far more likely if you simply decide that it will happen. Thinking about things, longing for things, having a vague ambition that you might quite like to achieve things - generally doesn't result in anything much happening at all.

So how is a decision different from just thinking about things, why will a decision, as opposed to vague thoughts make it happen? Well, it is all to do with your fabulous brain. It can perform all sorts of mindbogglingly complex tasks, but when it comes to multiple thoughts and desires, it might well need instruction; it needs specifics, and it needs focus.

A decision includes a specific set of instructions being sent to your brain. It also tells your brain that you have committed. You have decided; this specific set of things you want must be achieved. And armed with specifics, your brain will do all sorts of crazy things to make your wildest dreams come true - as long as you are specific about what your wildest dreams are. Your brain is like a magic genie - ask and it shall be received. Your brain will get you what you want, but first, you have to know what exactly you want, and how to ask for it. If you're generally quite miserable about being overweight, and it would be nice to be able to wear a bikini one day, then your poor brain is unsure what to do with that information. The fact that you are miserable being overweight does not help the brain know what you want instead. The bikini request is also a bit too vague; I know I can pop to the shops and buy a bikini in a size 20 but you won't see me lounging around the Costa Del Sol in one that size. So, you can see that your brain doesn't really have much to act on here. It doesn't know what you want. Worse, you don't sound all that serious about your desires either.

So first, we need to be clear about the ask. Personally, having spent my entire adult life pretending bikinis don't exist I genuinely have no desire to wear one, ever, so fitting into one, or even looking good in one for the five days I may get to spend near a beach each year really isn't something I'm all that bothered about. I do want to look good in the clothes I wear every day, though. I would like to pull on a pair of jeans and a jumper and not have to wear shapewear, or a long vest to cover up my bum. I would love to be able to buy a size 12 skirt and tuck a top into it and feel confident.

I do want to be a healthy weight. And whilst I have a cynical disdain for government guidelines on such matters, I do want my BMI to be under 25. I do! But I can be even more specific, I want to weigh 10 stones.

There, I've said it! I used to weigh 17 stones and at that point I would not, in my wildest dreams, have opted to decide to weigh less than 11 stones, as it felt too unrealistic. I will talk about goals later, but for now, it's more important to be specific than to be ambitious.

Here are the very specific decisions I have made about my own weight loss desires: I want to weigh 10 st. I want to fit easily into UK size 12 clothes or smaller. I want to feel confident in jeans and a top. I want to be able to wear tight dresses that show off my figure. Those are pretty exacting requests, aren't they? Now you know how to be specific, it's time to learn how to ask your brain to make things happen. I believe that by deciding to achieve your goals, you are effectively instructing your brain to do whatever it takes to ensure you achieve them.

The act of deciding is very powerful. Your brain now knows that this is a firm decision, you have spoken to your brain in a way that it can process the instruction. You can reinforce this decision every day, you can even reinforce this decision every single time you eat. As your brain hears your decision every day, it will start acting to help you implement it.

"I have decided I'll weigh 140 lb. I will fit easily into UK size 12 clothes or smaller. I will feel confident in jeans and a top. I will enjoy wearing tight dresses that show off my figure."

The decision is key, and I am pretty sure I would not have lost weight had I not decided to, had I simply wanted to, or tried to. Without deciding to I would not have been committed. By deciding, I told my brain what it was I wanted. I told it, and it listened. By making a decision, my brain had been instructed. It then just had to get on with it.

MAKING THE DECISION

Some people think there's no time like the present to decide to take action, whereas others might want to pick the perfect time and place. It's up to you. If you feel that making a decision would be better done on the top of a mountain, peering down upon the world, then fine. If you feel you just need to go and find a quiet moment sitting in the garden or your nearest park one morning, that's fine too. Whatever works for you. By the way, if you decide that you can only make the decision once you've done a bunch of other stuff then you're just delaying. You're deciding not to decide. You're deciding not to succeed.

I would pick a specific time when you can think about this carefully without being interrupted, so you can really savour your decision. I would also find a quiet space, outside where you can feel the air on your face; connect with nature.

When I decided to lose more weight to make sure I wasn't forever at the top of my healthy weight range, I sat in the middle of the park on a quiet morning. I spent a few minutes just relaxing, just sitting. I had written my decision down, much like I've shown you and then made my decision. Of course, had anyone appeared behind me and listened in they might have wondered what on earth I was on about, either that or thought I'd fallen over ill and needed help. But they didn't, and it was just me peacefully and successfully sharing my decision with the universe.

ACTIVITY

It's activity time again. This one is super fun and oh, so important. Turn to Activity 4 for help to craft your decision.

THE TYRANNY OF TRYING

For many of us who have tried to lose weight before and failed, or succeeded but then put the weight back on, we can blame our failure on indecision. We decided to try to lose weight rather than deciding to lose weight. Trying is the problem. Trying is pointless, I am afraid.

Unless you are committed, you are leaving room to say, 'I tried but it was too hard,' or 'I tried and lost a bit,' or whatever. Trying also implies it is super hard, that the reasonable expectation is for failure. By trying you are admitting that you probably won't lose weight. In fact, by trying you're basically setting yourself up to fail.

But deciding to lose weight, and actually then doing it on the other hand, is all powerful. Having decided to do something, you will make it happen. It simply will happen as the decision has been made. So, unless you decide to lose weight, you are deciding not to lose weight. It is that simple.

Don't fear the decision!

Deciding to do anything can be tricky. At the point of decision, you must acknowledge that it will take enormous effort, a huge amount of focus, and masses of self-love. You need to be ready to do it. To want it. To know it's possible (it is) and to know you can do it (you can).

Many of us run away at this point, I know I have in the past. I have read many self-help books over the years, to help me with one thing or another, and often there's a crunch point where you have to decide and commit, and this is because making decisions rather than 'trying and hoping for the best' is far more effective. I'd often get to the decision point and er, sort of skip that bit. I was subconsciously leaving the door open for failure.

Having had some weight loss success years ago, I used to think it was like flipping a switch. I'd talk happily about my weight loss switch. I'd flipped it on, and I was losing weight. The problem was, of course, that the switch could quite easily be flipped off. A decision on the other hand is final. It is a one way switch we flip ON. Forever.

Don't skip the decision.

ACTIVITY

This is the biggest decision you've made in a long time, possibly the biggest decision you have made ever. This is the most important activity in this book. You guessed it, it's time to make that decision. Look at Activity 5 for guidance on getting this right.

DEFINE YOUR GOALS

You are amazing. You can do anything. Yes, you can. You really can. I bet you have already done plenty of amazing stuff, and you're going to do plenty more utterly amazing things on your self-love and weight loss journey. So, remember this:

You can do anything.
You're going to achieve amazing things.
You are going to achieve anything you set your mind to (anything that you decide to).
You are going to decide to commit fully to losing weight.

When we commit to losing weight, we tend to have a specific goal in mind. But often, we aim low and begin with the expectation that we may not succeed. When I was 85 pounds overweight, my initial goal was to lose 20 pounds which is embarrassingly unambitious when you really think about it.

I never really believed I could reach a healthy weight, so there was no way that my aim was going to be to lose 85 pounds and I aimed low and settled on 20 pounds instead. But even that lowly aspiration was fragile from the start. I never really committed to it, I didn't share my goal with anyone else, and I didn't really decide on it either, as in the back of my mind, I knew I could scale down to 10 pounds or something even lower if my initial plan didn't work.

If you don't love yourself, you will inevitably set yourself unimpressive, shaky goals that you don't have the motivation to achieve. Without loving yourself, you lack the self-assurance that you will achieve whatever you set out to do. When you're operating at this level, goals become rather pointless rather quickly.

Beautiful, Happy, Awesome Goals

I have worked in at least two businesses that used the term "BHAG" to describe business goals. In these businesses, BHAG meant "Big Hairy Audacious Goals" - which, well, is self-explanatory. However, in most businesses the ability to set, let alone achieve anything audacious is limited, and any hairiness is dismissed as being too risky. In reality, the BHAGs that I encountered were more MAUGs - Medium, Achievable, Unexciting Goals. No sort of goals at all.

Some people say that goals that are not 'stretchy', as in that they don't take you outside of your comfort zone, aren't goals at all. I think that's true, and, as achieving any sort of weight loss will definitely take you out of your comfort zone, your goal will absolutely be a stretchy goal. When deciding to create a brand new you, it's essential that you are fully signed up to the process. Now I'm going to help you set, achieve, and use goals in a new way. I've designed a new type of BHAG - the Beautiful, Happy, Awesome Goal, and it works like this. Your goal must be:

Beautiful - It must come from a position of love and be something you want to do for yourself purely because you're someone you really love and think of as amazing.

Happy - It must make you feel happy, and not worried that you can't achieve it. This goal can't be something you wouldn't tell someone else about, and it certainly can't be unambitious.

Awesome - It must be awesome. Not low-balled. Awesome.

Goals Build

If you are right at the beginning of your weight loss journey and you have any sort of serious weight to lose you are unlikely to want to start with a massive goal. That's okay but that's not to say your goal should be feeble. Remember it should be awesome, but it is absolutely fine to treat the goal-setting exercise as your chance to set your *first* goal.

When you love yourself, and when you've made your decision to lose weight and when you've set your BHAG, achieving this goal will be easy. And then you'll need another one. Another one?

Yes, you heard right.

Let's say your first goal is to lose 10 pounds. You embark on the mission and lose the 10 pounds with ease. At this point, you have proven to yourself that you can do amazing things and you'll know you can achieve another, bigger goal. Maybe your next goal is to lose 20 pounds, or to fit into a certain pair of jeans. As you achieve each amazing goal, you can create another, more ambitious one. In this way, your goals build over time and what starts out relatively small - losing five, seven or 10 pounds, can soon turn into 'lose 20 pounds' or 'lose 50 pounds' or more. By setting, achieving, and building on your goals, you're proving to yourself that you can achieve amazing things regularly.

The alternative is starting with a massive 85-pound sized goal and not actually achieving that for a very long time. It's so far away, so hard, and you don't get the fuzzy feeling you get when you smash through your goals regularly with awesome style.

There's no such thing as 'perfect'

Now before you go off to define a goal like 'I'm gonna look great in a shocking pink bikini' or 'I'm gonna be a model', I want to offer a word of caution. We have talked about how a goal should be awesome - and yes, that means transformational. When ensuring your goal is awesome, make it big enough, ambitious enough, and enough of a transition from where you are today. But and this is a big but… don't aspire for perfect.

I hate perfect. I really do. I hate it with a passion. I hate it for so many reasons.

Firstly, perfect is a myth. Perfect does not exist. There simply is no such thing as perfect. What is perfect to you will not be perfect to someone else. It's subjective; no two people will agree on perfection.

Secondly, perfect is competitive. For you, or for anyone else. If perfect did exist it would represent the best ever possible state. To be perfect, you would need to be the very best, better than all the rest. Being the best in the world at something is a tall order. Whether you could be the best or not, when you have self love on your side you simply don't need to compete.

Thirdly, perfect is dull. We are all human and by our nature as humans, we are all brilliantly imperfect. It is our differences and quirks that make us who we are, that make us attractive to people.

Fourthly, perfect is fake. Visions of perfect we may see from A-list stars to C-list celebs, to wannabe influencers are not all what they seem. You know what I mean. I am not suggesting all images are photoshopped or are fakes, but you don't need to benchmark yourself against people, images or lifestyles that are staged.

Fifthly, perfect is impossible. For most of us, 'perfect' is simply not available.   If your goal is to shift a (proverbial or otherwise) ton of weight, it is extremely unlikely your body will bounce back to being super skinny, or that you won't have any loose skin, or that your shape will be flattered by a skimpy bikini.

You do need a dash of realism here. It is extremely exciting to fit into smaller clothes, and to imagine that one day a trip to a beach won't be a torturous experience, but it is also important to accept any imperfections you will still have, and to learn to love yourself in your imperfect state. It is highly unlikely anyone can go from being overweight to having the body of a supermodel. And you should absolutely be entirely okay with that.

Finally, and most importantly, you don't need perfect. When you love yourself, you love yourself, and that's enough.

ACTIVITY

Let's set some goals. Check out Activity 6 for help with goal setting.

CREATE THE RIGHT MINDSET RECAP

So now you're starting to learn about how to create the right mindset for self-love and weightloss. In this section I've talked about the need to start by defining your whys so that you truly know why you're on this journey. You have to know why you're doing something, why you're really doing something to really be able to do it.

I've also talked about affirmations and their role in helping you to remind yourself why you're here and how awesome you are every day. Affirmations will be your guiding light. You'll learn to really enjoy them even if they do feel a little strange at first; having fun with them and making them uniquely personal always helps. Goals are important too and the LYALW method asks you to define Beautiful, Happy, Awesome Goals that can build over time.

The most important thing in this section for me though is stop trying! Yes, stop trying; simply decide and then do.

Food is Your Friend

I want to reassure you that you can eat whatever you like with this method. However, you might at this point be worried I'm gonna insist on limiting you to a thousand calories a day. Well, no, I'm not going to do that. You can eat whatever you like, you can eat bread, and cake and ice cream if that's what you really want and consider to be beautiful food. You can eat it when you're hungry and eat as much of it as you like until you're full.

So, if you can eat whatever you like whenever you like, what's the catch? How does this help you to lose weight if you're just eating what you eat right now?

The 'catch' is that loving the food you eat, is not eating how you eat now. How you eat now is not loving, or joyous, or enjoyable. And if you were to tell me you really loved cake, I'm afraid I'd have to say, 'I don't think you really do'.

Be honest with yourself. Do you really love shovelling in a whole 600 or so calories of cake, biscuits, or crisps only to feel hungry and miserable 30 minutes later?

Food Myths

People who put on weight generally have a poor relationship with food. You may think you love what you are eating simply because the advertising industry or the people around you have told you that you love these foods. You have been repeatedly told that you just can't get enough pizza, that eating high-calorie, high-carb burger meals is a fun way to spend time with your family, and that it's completely natural for women to indulge in endless chocolate to get through a tough day, and that everyone (and I mean everyone) is addicted to caffeine just to get as far as work. You'd think families ate every meal at McDonald's, that all women had boxes of chocolate on an Amazon Dash button or that literally no one drank decaf.

The people who create these myths work in advertising or marketing and get paid to help massive corporations sell more of their cheap-to-produce, high profit margin foods. These advertising types are creative and want to help inspire you to buy something. They will very cleverly align certain products to specific emotions and will use behavioural science to tap into your subconscious mind.

Advertising seeks to normalise certain bad behaviours so that you feel it's okay, and perfectly normal to eat a whole 'stuffed crust' pepperoni to yourself plus a side of garlic bread simply because it is too irresistible to resist. No one can resist. Good God, you'd think we could take over governments or win wars simply by rocking up with a pizza and rendering people completely defenceless. I shouldn't really joke as this is a serious issue. This is the same advertising industry that made kids think smoking was cool, or that drinking vodka shots is a great idea. We shouldn't think that's okay today, and we certainly won't think peddling cheap, unsustaining foods is okay in a few years' time either.

I can hear you thinking that now I'm suddenly going to introduce a food ban. Well, no foods are forbidden on the LYALW method, but I do want you to think very carefully about the foods you choose to eat. As you can probably tell, I feel incredibly angry about the fact that that the foods that do us the least good are sold to us as the foods that are the most delicious, the foods that are hard to do without. But are they really that amazing? Or have we just been conditioned to think that they are? I think, to be honest, we've just been told a lie, a lie that we can't do without these foods, so that we think we're addicted to them when we're not.

I am not even suggesting you do without these foods, but I would like you to learn more about why we think certain foods are so amazing. True, a pizza slice, baked just right with warming melted cheese and a few jalapeños is tasty, but so are a lot of other things. It's just a sad fact that there aren't teams of advertising strategists and creatives all staying up late (and they do stay up late) working out how to use behavioural science to get you to think you can't do without foods that would be really good for you.

There is no team of ad execs tearing their hair out dreaming up a new way to get you hooked on tomatoes, or salmon, or strawberries or chamomile tea. There may well be a lot of money in these foods, but not nearly as much money as there is in pizza, burgers, crisps, biscuits and cookies, and breakfast cereal. There are big companies involved in the production of these foods with big brand names. There's an eye-watering amount of money at stake.

Advertisers want you to think something is tasty; that it's decadent. Hell, they even want you to feel that it's a little bit bad for you, so you'll really want it. Ultimately, pizza is just bread and cheese with a little flavour thrown in. It is low in nutrients, will fill you up, but it makes you hungry for more later because it doesn't have the right nutrients to satisfy you - it simply doesn't deliver what your body needs.

So why are we sold the idea that we should be hooked on food like pizza, crisps, burgers, biscuits, cake, bread, and sweets?

Because they are cheap as, well, chips! They require the cheapest processed flour and sugar to make, and often, they contain hardly any protein or fruit or vegetables. These foods are low in nutrients. They are cheap to make in factories, dark kitchens, or takeaway houses by lowly paid workers and they're sold to you as a lifestyle choice, as convenient, indulgent, even luxurious treats.

Brands, restaurant chains, and global businesses need you to buy and eat these foods. They need you to buy and eat these foods because they can make them cheaply and sell them to you with a high markup. There's profit in these foods; lots of profit. One of the most famous pizza delivery businesses took over $4 billion in revenues in 2020[6]. So, you see, there are literally billions of pounds to be made from selling cheap food. And to sell billions of pounds worth of cheap food, these businesses need you to absolutely believe that you can't get enough of these items, that you're already hooked, and that resistance is futile.

Before we were duped into having to eat certain foods, which we were told were so delicious, so indulgent and that we somehow deserved to treat ourselves to, we had very different ideas about food. As a society, we used to believe in 'a balanced diet', we used to advocate 'three square meals' – which were often a balanced meal of 'meat and two veg'. Since when did junk food contain meat, or protein, or veg? It is only recently that we have come to think that eating large amounts of junk is normal, something we just must do. In the 1970s, before we were so saturated with food advertising, we may have enjoyed the odd biscuit, the odd pizza even, but empty carbs were not rammed down our throats so much. People were smaller: far fewer people were overweight or obese.

This is a fact you should take on board – worldwide obesity has nearly tripled since 1975[7].

---

[6] https://www.statista.com/statistics/207133/revenue-of-dominos-pizza/

[7] https://www.worldobesity.org/about/about-obesity/prevalence-of-obesity

Knowing that most of your food favourites are cheap to make, contain little nutritional value, and are the key profit drivers for large corporations – are they still the kind of thing you want to feed the person you love the most in the world?

I doubt it. When people have babies, most parents buy into another advertising message – and that is that their newborn is the most precious thing in the world and deserves to eat healthily. Parents buy endless plastic pouches of mushed up vegetables because they're sold as organic. That makes them nutritious, right?

Don't worry, I am just as guilty of buying those little pouches of pre-mushed vegetables as you are. If I'd just boiled some potato and carrots and not put salt in, I could have fed my child the same thing for a fraction of the cost. We are all susceptible to advertising and I don't expect you to be able to ignore or erase decades of powerful messaging; the conditioning that's led you to hold your current beliefs about food. We have all been manipulated. But now it's time to make a stand – really ask yourself what you like to eat, and what foods truly make you feel amazing.

The first step in undoing years of conditioning, of being made to believe that you really want a heavy stodgy pizza (remember, it's just bread with cheese on the top) is to question it. Just question it. When you see an advert for pizza, instead of simply craving one, just ask yourself:

Is this what I really want?
Is this going to make me feel great?
Is this going to sustain me?
Why do I want this?
Do I want this because I have just seen an ad for it?
What is the ad telling me?
Is the ad telling me that even though I know this food is not great for me, won't sustain me, and will likely make me feel miserable, everyone else is eating this food, so why am I so special, why should I do anything different?

Well, get this: you are special. Remember you're the person you love most (or joint most) in the world. You deserve to be treated well, with respect and care. You deserve to be fed delicious, sustaining, nutritious, gorgeous foods that make you feel great about yourself. So how do you find the good stuff when you're used to the junk? How do you start eating the healthy food, when you still believe the BS about the junk food? I don't expect you to fully get this yet, or to fully agree with me right now. I expect there will be some dissent, worry, concern, or rebellion even. Don't be put off by this, resistance is entirely normal.

If you're now assuming that I'm telling you that all the food you love is junk and should be avoided, and that this really is just another diet, then you're wrong. Remember you can eat what you want to eat. You can eat pizza, you can eat chocolate, you can eat crisps, or biscuits if that's what you want, as long as you eat it consciously, and you enjoy every single mouthful incredibly slowly. You can eat those foods, but I want you to start thinking more about the types of foods you choose to eat. The types of foods that attract you.

LOVE WHAT YOU EAT

Never in a million years are you going to see ads on television or online, or on those glossy leaflets that come through the door for a poached salmon salad, or for tomatoes, or omelettes, or naked keto cheeseburgers, or a bowl of cherries, but these are all delicious foods. Never are you going to see an advert for a Chicken Madras with cauliflower rice, or an ad for chaffles - for the uninitiated, chaffles are like waffles but are made with egg and cheese and are low-carb friendly.

Whilst I am not advocating the keto diet, I like many of its principles, it just isn't for me. So chaffles, cauliflower rice (rice made from cauliflower as a low/no carb alternative - eat as much as you like). Tomatoes and cherries probably aren't high up in your mind as something you ought to desire. But they easily could be.

I don't mean to be patronising by assuming that you are someone who falls for advertising – but the truth is, we all do. We all think we know pizza tastes amazing whereas tomatoes are just tomatoes. But just because certain foods aren't heavily advertised doesn't mean that they aren't delicious. Far from it, the fact that a food is not really advertised all that much is way more likely to mean that this specific food is expensive, and that there's not much profit in it. Companies make more profit when you eat cheap food, so it makes sense that they don't want you to buy food that's more expensive to make.

If we extrapolate this argument, we may well have to face the awful truth that giant corporations get richer as we all get fatter. Is that okay? What do you think? Is that okay for the person you love most in the world? Is that okay for you? Even if the corporations don't want us to be fat, they certainly don't have our best interests at heart. And that's okay, we can't and shouldn't rely on others to make sure we're healthy, we have our own free will and we need to use it.

I realised there was some Grade A crap going on around food advertising early on in my weight loss journey, I was researching baby foods as my daughter was coming up to six months old. I felt that insane love only parents feel where they'd do anything to find the perfect food for their child and that feeding them anything except the best could basically mean the child would end up in the gutter by age 11.

I started to question things. I started to question myself. During my pregnancy I had been compelled to enter any McDonald's restaurant I saw and eat a Quarter Pounder® with Cheese Meal whatever time of day it was, and I had these indulgences alongside my 'regular' oversized meals. I blamed pregnancy, and to be fair, this wasn't a normal way to eat, even for me. It felt like my body was urging me to eat all the food I could find.

But by the time my daughter was ready to go onto solids, I was done with deluding myself and I had started listening to my body more. It had been through a lot; carrying a child when you're already significantly overweight is not easy. I was thinking about what to feed my baby, so it made sense to also think about my own food. We went healthy. The supermarket deliveries suddenly had more veg in them, and fruit - although I had never actually liked fruit before. Now I love bananas, apples, cherries, and raspberries. I am still not sure what all the fuss is about with strawberries, but you can't have it all. Before I lost weight, I now realise it was not a case of me not liking fruit, rather, I just never ate it, as I always ate other types of sweet foods. I ate chocolate, puddings, ice cream, fancy ice cream, ice cream with biscuit dough shoved into it, as if eating ice cream was not quite enough on its own.

So, you see, it is possible to learn to like new foods. It is also possible to start to like foods you may love a little less, and it is possible to dislike foods that you once loved. Over time, with self-love on your side, you'll be able to question yourself more. Do you really want that pizza? And the garlic bread side? Or would you like to try something else?

Not all calories are created equal

These days, I mainly stay away from carbs, however, I do occasionally eat pizza, and there's nothing wrong with that - occasionally eating a little pizza is okay but eating a lot of pizza often is a totally different proposition. And the big problem with that is not that a large stuffed crust pepperoni pizza with extra cheese has a gazillion calories, is super heavy and makes you bloated, or that overeating stretches your stomach, so you get used to needing more food, or that it is high in salt, and low in vitamins. No, that's not the problem. The problem is also not that it is cheap food, that you've overpaid for and that you're lining the pockets of the already wealthy shareholders of big corporations. That's also not the problem. The problem is not that it was made without much care for the environment and might contain intensively farmed pork from pigs that have not been treated all that well, and cheese from cows raised on land where forests used to grow. Nope, that's not the problem. Nor is the issue that carbs give you a high that quickly dissipates and leads you to want to load up on yet more carbs very soon afterwards. The main problem isn't that it comes in a giant, environmentally unfriendly, cardboard box. Nor that the delivery driver who brought it to you was paid minimum wage on a 'zero hours contract'. Not that. Although that is a very real problem.

The even bigger problem for you of overeating lots of pizza is that it tells you that you don't really care about you. It is a very loud and clear message that you don't really love yourself all that much. Where has your guardian angel or your superhero gone? Are they off on a lunch break? Who's got your back? Who's treating you right? Stuffing yourself with pizza isn't what you'd do for the person you love most in the world, is it? If you have real self-love, it isn't what you should want for yourself.

Also, eating like this really isn't what everyone is doing, despite what the advertisers want you to believe. They think that shoving a leaflet through your letter box with a glossy picture of a pizza slices dripping in melting cheese will make it okay, normalise it, and make you think that you are not alone. If you're ordering one, so are other people, maybe other people in your street, maybe your next-door neighbour. Everyone's at it, so it's okay. Or at least that's what you like to tell yourself, isn't it?

When you have self-love on your side and you're losing weight it's unlikely you'll want to order pizza. It's also unlikely that you'll never eat pizza again. But you'll find a happy medium whereby you eat pizza when you really want it and you know it's what's right for you at that time, you'll eat it slowly and really enjoy it and because you've eaten it slowly and consciously, you'll stop after a small amount. You really will be able to take it or leave it. You will – however unlikely that might seem to you today.

Take your Time

Also, and here's the bizarre thing: overeating masses of junk food simply isn't what people who really care about themselves do. Do you have a thin mate who takes their time over food, who can be around any amount of any food and just simply slowly eat a bit then stop? Even if it was never ending? Even if it was free?

I have one such friend. This friend used to really perplex me as he would often take a painfully long time to prepare a meal. He'd then sit and 'get around to' eating it at some point later - way after he'd finished slowly making it. When he did get around to eating it, he'd eat it really slowly. Then he'd leave some!!! OMG, it was as if he wasn't totally compelled to stuff his face. If presented with something junky he would have some, but maybe just one piece of pizza, or maybe two, but one at a time. He'd eat pizza slowly. He'd put it down between bites. It was often irritating as it put everyone else to shame. This wasn't some bizarre spiritual ritual that was confusing and shaming, no, this was just something called normal eating.

Funnily enough, without all the brainwashing from advertising, humans instinctively think about what they eat, and they eat it slowly to enjoy it. Then, because they know there'll be more when they need it, they stop eating. Sometimes before their plates are empty! Heavens above. We can learn a lot from our slow eating friends. They eat consciously, and when you eat consciously, you can indeed eat what you like, because you think about it. Because you're conscious around food.

I've talked, and perhaps ranted about foods we think we love but don't; foods that we may think we love but that certainly don't love us back in return. But what about good food, food we really do love? The Love Yourself and Lose Weight method is not about disliking food, it is instead all about loving food, so let's talk about how to love what you eat.

Consciousness is key. Whatever situation you find yourself in; be it staring into your fridge with grumbling hunger pangs, reading the menu in your favourite restaurant, or filling your trolley up in the supermarket: THINK. Just think about what you choose at every choice. Ask yourself:
Is this what I really want?

Do I want this because I've just seen an advert for it?
Why do I want this?
Is this going to sustain me?
Is this going to make me feel great?
How amazing is this going to make me feel?
Is this what I'd choose for someone I really love?

Food is hugely important to us; it sustains us, it helps us thrive. It can make us feel amazing, it can be supremely enjoyable. Eating wonderful, healthy, gorgeous, tasty, beautiful food can give you such a buzz. If you're not used to getting a buzz from uplifting food, this is a skill you can learn. It may not be instant, but you will get there in time.

The LYALW method is not a diet because I am not telling you what to eat, but I am telling you how to eat; it's an important distinction and vital to understand that these are two very different things. When you change what you eat by going on a diet, it is instant. You follow the prescribed diet - you have instantly changed what you eat. If you follow the diet, you will succeed. Diets are of course impossible to follow because no one wants to eat what someone else tells them to for the rest of their lives. You are an individual and you need to exercise your own free will over what you eat every day.

Changing how you eat, on the other hand, is not instant, it takes longer, and it takes a lot more effort from you. You will need to think about how you eat, whereas a diet entirely prescribes your intake, and takes you and your free will out of the picture.

Let's be honest here, weight gain normally comes from overeating, doesn't it? And overeating is generally the result of not being mindful about what you are eating. If you just change what you eat but never change how you eat, losing weight will be hard. Sure, you will create a calorie deficit and shift some of those pounds, but you'll be working against what your body and your mind are telling you to do. That's why diets are hard to stick to. You have a list of what to eat but your mind and body wants something else.

When you change how you eat on the other hand, you can start with a few small changes and build more in later. There's no requirement to change everything about how you think about food on day one. How you eat covers all aspects of your food choices and eating preferences, such as:

- Which food you're naturally drawn to.
- Which food you try.
- Which food you buy.
- How much you make.
- How much you serve.

- How slowly you eat.
- How much you savour your food.
- How much you leave on your plate.
- How much you throw away.

I can't and shouldn't prescribe any of this. There's a right way to eat for you to sustain a healthy weight. There's also a right way to eat for you that will mean you lose weight, and thankfully, there's a right way for you to eat that will mean you lose weight whilst still thoroughly enjoying the food you eat.

Changing how you eat could take years. (If I'm honest, it has for me). Nobody goes from being a fan of junk food one evening and wakes up as someone who thinks of their body as a temple the next. When you change how you eat, you must change how your mind works, as opposed to just the foods you put in your mouth. I like to think about it as learning how to eat like a thin person.

Eat Consciously

If I ever think about what it would be like to be in prison (I don't do this often), I think one of the worst elements would be not being in control of what you eat. You and I are lucky enough to have choices about what we eat, and even if we're overweight, we should grab onto that fundamental right - as opposed to asking someone else we've never met to tell us what we must eat. Changing how you eat is the key to achieving your weight loss goals.

ACTIVITY

Consciousness is key. Look at Activity 7 for handy tips to check whether what you think you want to eat is really what you want to eat.

As I learned to love myself, I recognised that how I ate was not appropriate for someone who loved herself. I was eating like someone who really didn't care about myself very much, so I started experimenting with different ways of eating, and I learned an awful lot about my attitudes towards food along the way.

Losing weight is not just about the food you eat. As we've discussed, you first need to identify and bring the good YOU to the table; you know, the version of you who acts like your very own fairy godmother, or superhero. Once they have shown up to the party, the food bit will be way easier as they'll do their bit to keep you on track.

You need to see bad food for what it really is – self-harm on a plate. Instead of focusing on the idea that you can't have cake, be grateful that you have started to see what cake is really like. Once you make this shift in your thinking, you might begin to wonder how you were ever brainwashed into liking cake for so long.

Remember all the lies you have been told about how hard it is to lose weight. The biggest lie I've been told is that to lose fat you can't eat fat. We all know that one is simply incorrect, but we still see it everywhere. I know I've certainly lost weight eating a diet that included butter, cheese and full fat yoghurt, and unashamedly enjoyed these foods while dropping the pounds.

LOVE YOURSELF & LOSE WEIGHT

LYALW RULES

There are rules to the LYALW method, but they are rules that work for you, and they won't necessarily work for anyone else. Losing weight is a very personal thing, and that's how it should be. Your body is your body, and what works for someone else with a different body shape, a different amount of weight to lose, a different metabolism and different reactions to food is not going to work in the same way for you.

Far from being alarming, this is good news. Don't worry! There's no simple one size fits all plan here; instead, you get to create your own programme that is completely right for you. At the risk of contradicting myself, there are, of course, some basic rules that work for everyone. My rules are the rules of someone with 40 odd years of experience of eating food and are not those of a nutritionist. Mine are the rules of someone who needed to and attempted to lose weight and who tried various 'diets' or weight loss food plans.

Over the years, I have tried the Keto diet, Atkins, Weight Watchers, general starvation, popping diet pills, and even some nonsense that involved cottage cheese and something awful called quark. From all this unsuccessful experience, I have learned so much about why diets don't work, which foods are good or bad for me, and what and how to eat to lose weight. I have learned this through experimentation and importantly through listening to my body. Whilst I don't want to tell you specifically what to eat, there are food groups, and some are better for you than others. Specifically, it is important to note that:

- Sugar is bad.
- Carbs are bad (carbs are sugar).
- Alcohol is bad (alcohol is sugar and it also makes you do silly things and feel less than impressed with yourself the next day).
- Protein is good.
- Fat is good (to varying degrees).
- Low fat diets are not all that.
- Low fat, high carb diets are terrible.

Low fat diets are awful. They're terrible because they starve you of the things that your body needs, and they often substitute fat for sugar. In most cases, low fat equals high sugar. Any diet is bad that expects you to eliminate cheese, milk, meat, and oily fish and to replace them with empty carbs such as pasta, and granola etc.

Carbs are bad. Carbs are bad. Carbs are bad. I can't say it enough. Or at least empty carbs are bad for me, and might just be bad for you too.

I am not advocating a super-low-carb, high-fat diet like keto although I know keto works for lots of people. I am simply advising that you cut down on carbs A LOT. White rice, pasta or bread are basically just as 'bad for you' as cake. You can have pasta, rice, and bread, but in small amounts. You can have cake in small amounts too. But it's important to remember that most carbs are poor quality foods because they don't nourish you; they are empty calories, and they keep you craving more carbs. In my mind, carbs can be as bad for some people as cigarettes are for us all - and are just as addictive.

It is vitally important that as you move forward on your weight loss journey that you listen to your body. If you eat consciously and carefully, and really think about what and how you eat, you will make conscious choices. If you base your food choices on the rules above, you will be eating a lower carb, higher protein diet. You can experiment with the fats, protein and fibre you eat. You can also experiment with carbs. If you are a bread lover, this may be hard to cut out. I loved rice, and for a long time, I thought I could never do without it. But I did need to do without it to lose masses of weight. I still ate a little bit of it though.

Eating food that you love is very important. You love yourself so it is vital you fill your body with lovely healthy food. As you learn to love yourself more and to eat consciously you will learn to understand the great joy that you can get from eating well. You must eat consciously to start to make a change, to embed the change as a habit and to make sure you keep making the right choices every day - the choices you'd make for someone you love the most in the world. Here's how to stay on track with conscious eating:

Eat with love: Every time you eat, you're going to stop and also feed yourself love. This ensures that you remember that you love yourself several times a day. It also slows down your eating, as you consider yourself for a moment before you start eating. What I mean by 'eat with love' is that when you eat, remind yourself that you love you. Say your affirmations or your whys in your head each time you eat.

Listen to your body: Chose what you want to eat - and listen to what your body is telling you. Cravings serve a purpose: they give your body the nutrients it needs.

Eat pretty: Feed yourself beautiful, life sustaining, healthy food, the kind you would give to the person who you love most in the whole world. Before selecting food either at home, in the supermarket, or whilst eating out, ask yourself whether what you're about to eat is what you would choose for your favourite person in your world. If it passes that test you can go ahead. Make sure it looks good too.

Drink with love: Always drink a glass of water before you eat. Often when you feel hunger, you are actually thirsty, so the water will quench your thirst. It will fill you up, so you'll want to eat less. And most importantly, this will slow you down, and will stop you from launching straight into the eating part. By drinking a glass of water, you'll take a moment to think, to remind yourself of your whys and you will remember to eat slowly.

Eat slowly: Eat really slowly. Think about your whys and as you eat, savour every mouthful, enjoy the beautiful food.

Stop eating: Stopping eating when you're full is not really a trick, at least not for people who don't struggle with their weight, but it is a trick for those of us who do. Many of us don't stop when we're full. We don't stop when we're full because we don't notice we're full as we're too busy shovelling. By slowing down our eating we will notice the feeling of being full, or stuffed, more quickly.

As soon as you start to feel full, just stop eating. When I learned to do this, I found it quite hard, as I was so used to simply keeping going; I'd keep going until the plate was empty. If you are worried about stopping eating when you think you're full, or as you start to get full, don't worry. You can stop, then have a think about how you feel, how hungry you feel, and if you feel hungry you can eat more. Stopping eating was difficult for me for a while until I learned to feel that I was in control, and I could stop or start as I desired if I was hungry.

This list might look like a lot to remember. At first, it is important to follow the steps and to take these instructions seriously. Remember too that if you don't create self-love, you will find it hard to eat well, so it won't work. If you do the self-love part but then wolf down giant portions without slowing down and really thinking about what you are doing to your body, you probably won't manage to lose weight either. If I can give you one piece of advice about how to achieve happiness and weight loss, it's this:

Losing weight is about changing your mind to change your body. It is about food but not just about food. Focus on loving yourself enough to change how you eat.

ACTIVITY

Check out Activity 8 to help you think about the foods that truly make you happy.

FOOD IS YOUR FRIEND RECAP

So you see we're all rather brainwashed about food, but holding onto our old beliefs isn't going to help us to make a change. We all need to think critically every time we make choices about food - when we shop, go out, cook and eat. Considering how food makes us feel and whether it's truly the food we'd give the person we love most in the world can help us make the right choices every time, or at least, more often than not! The LYALW method has some rules to eat by that you can adapt to suit your circumstances, that you can use to create the perfect non-diet for you.

Love Moving

Every morning, the first thing I do is to get myself running around the park for at least two miles. And the strange thing is that I don't do this because I feel I have to – I do it for fun. Even as I write these words, you have no idea how ridiculous they still sound to me, because as someone who spent many years as a Size 18-20 coach potato, I can't quite believe how much I have changed.

But before you get scared off, and assume I'm telling you to run around every morning in the dark and cold, I'm not.

Don't worry you don't need to do this. Unless you want to, that is. But what is really important for your weight loss journey is to start enjoying moving every day. It doesn't matter how far or fast you run or walk, or which type of fancy Pilates you do, or whether you know what HIIT is, or whether you cycle to get to places or cycle in your living room. No, what is important is that you move your body. Even just a bit. Even just a tiny bit.

Exercise will be your friend, but I am aware that maybe exercise hasn't been your friend so far. Perhaps exercise has even been your enemy. Perhaps exercise is simply something that you've never tried, that you feel doesn't work for you. Maybe exercise is something that other people do; something that only thin people do. Well, exercise is something that people do; that thin people do, that fat people do, that people who are successful at losing weight do. And whether you currently do Zumba twice a week or whether the last time you ran was at the age of 16 when a vindictive PE teacher made everyone run a 'whole' mile at school - exercise in some form will help you to lose weight.

Why does exercise help people to lose weight? Okay, okay, so we ain't stupid, right? We all know that exercise is good for us. I don't really need to spell it out, do I? Maybe, I do.

False Beliefs

I was definitely someone who considered herself to be in the 'not stupid' category. I did all sorts of fancy work helping businesses to adopt new technology. I even had a degree in the Arts. I was creative and clever, and in many ways, successful. But when it came to moving my body, well, I was a total moron. I knew nothing about it. Worse than knowing nothing about it, I had formed the most incredibly stupid beliefs about exercise – that it would hurt, was horribly boring and was something that dull people did that I simply didn't need.

Exercise was not something that played a major part in my upbringing. Whilst it wasn't explicitly frowned upon, it wasn't exactly encouraged either. We went swimming, but this was seen as a life skill rather than a way to keep fit. There was the odd bit of aerobics going on amongst my family as I grew up in the 80s, but I suspect the attraction was more likely the pastel Dash tracksuits rather than the exercise itself.

We owned an elaborate clothes horse which you could also sit on and turn pedals with your legs. I may even have seen family members attempt to push the pedals around once or twice, but usually it just displayed the clothes that had been flung at it, or it sat lonely in the spare bedroom. Cars on the other hand were great.

Cars were for getting you to where you were going; not walking. Walking was something people who owned wellies did. We did not walk. People who owned dogs walked. We did not own a dog. If anyone suggested going for a walk, they'd be met with indignation as if they'd asked us to lug all their furniture up a mountain. So, I grew up believing that moving my body, apart from to and from a car and around some shops, was generally not all that exciting or necessary.

Exercise was also not something I did much of at school either. The only sport me and my friends were really good at was the sport of avoiding PE lessons. Apart from the usual excuse of having our period, we concocted all sorts of ludicrous excuses to avoid hockey, running and athletics. I was so well-known for my excuses that a teacher once made me complete a gymnastics class even though I complained of a severe pain in my foot. We had been asked to 'fly through the air' and having landed badly I had broken my metatarsal.

Netball was weirdly a different story for me as I quite liked it. To be honest though, there's' not much running involved and if you catch the ball, you basically have to stand still with it. Sorry netballers, but it just seemed much easier and way less terrible than hockey! Netball, though, was something I even did outside of school, and I even played for my county team, until I was about 16 and discovered that hanging around the town centre with boys was more fun.

So, you see, exercise, apart from my short-lived flirtation with netball, was not something I liked, not something I did and not something I took into adulthood. The sad thing is that I know that there are millions of people like me who did a little exercise when we were young under duress, but as we got older, we wouldn't have been seen dead in a gym.

Yet despite my absolute reluctance to get moving, I always knew that exercise was good for me, but I just couldn't get past my entrenched beliefs that it was unpleasant, it was hard, and really, pretty thankless.

But I still knew it was a good thing to do (in theory). I also knew of all these other people who thought it was amazing and couldn't get enough of it. Some of them thought it was so good that they did it regularly and voluntarily, but I was never one of them. Quite simply, I had convinced myself that exercise was something I hated, so I gave it a miss, which looking back now, seems like an awful shame. I regret not having challenged my beliefs about exercise before I did. I could have lost weight earlier. More likely I would never have put on the weight, or at least not put so much weight on.

The Benefits of Exercise

What is it about exercise that makes it so good for us? Well, there's plenty of science that proves exercise is good for us. I'm not a scientist and I don't want to make any dodgy claims but from my own experience alone, I know that:

- It burns calories - so helps to achieve a calorie deficit (which speeds up weight loss)
- It speeds up your metabolism - so helps you to digest and process food (which helps with weight loss)
- It helps your body to burn the fat first (which helps with weight loss)
- It builds muscle (which makes exercise easier and helps with weight loss)
- It helps you to feel less tired - so you have more energy to move more (which helps with weight loss)
- If you're doing cardio, your heart and lungs gets healthier (which might make you live longer)

And that's just physically. There are a whole lot of emotional benefits too:

- It gives you an endorphin rush (which makes you feel good)

- It makes you look better more quickly (which makes you feel good)
- It gets easier over time, so you get better at it, so you feel a sense of achievement (which makes you feel good)
- You get in a sort of meditative state (or I do anyway) which chills you out for the day
- You get to feel smug knowing you've done a workout or even more smug if you can get it done before 8am (which makes you feel great)

OMG, you're telling me this exercise gig is something to be enjoyed? Yep, sorry, I was wrong. I was so wrong, I mean I was right at the time; running around a hockey pitch in zero degrees wearing a tiny skirt with freezing legs, which your so-called friends are attempting to hit with wooden sticks is not enjoyable. Why would anyone do that? But my old beliefs about other forms of exercise were absolutely, entirely, utterly wrong.

It's okay to be wrong by the way, it's better to be wrong and change your mind than it is to be that person forever. There's no need to keep clinging onto old beliefs if they no longer serve you.

So, we've established that we believe the things we've been told, even if they are other people's beliefs and not our own. We create our own new beliefs by telling ourselves new things. We can easily create a world for ourselves in which exercise is bad and is something we'd never do, never be able to do, and most certainly would never, ever enjoy. We can also break this world down, admit we may be wrong, or at least that we may not be right, or at the very least, that it's worth giving it a go to see.

It's not just about food

The benefits of exercise are huge but the exercise itself need not be. I believe that moving your body is a vital part of a successful weight loss method. Attempting to lose weight without any exercise is like baking a cake without flour; it is possible, but the results are just a bit unpredictable. If you attempt to achieve a calorie deficit alone, you will lose weight, but the exercise bit helps you achieve your calorie deficit more quickly, speeds up your metabolism, tones your body, makes you look great and generally quickens the weight loss whilst giving you endorphins, a sense of achievement and of course, total smugness.

Which type of exercise you do is up to you. I have talked about the torturous sports they make you play in school because they hate you. Don't do those things. They will always be awful and it's okay that you will never do those things again. I am never, ever going to play hockey and I am very comfortable with that. I promise that on my death bed I won't be telling anyone that I wished I'd played more hockey. Times change however, and since I was at school, they've invented new types of exercise.

WHAAAT!!??! New types of exercise? Yes, and some of them are not terrible. Some of them are fun. You might even like some of them. There is so much out there that we've never tried, certainly many, many things I've never tried and really should, there's bound to be something that's right for you. Now many types of exercise involve going somewhere to work out or to do a class. Don't be put off by this. Those evil places they call gyms are not all so evil. Lots more people have plucked up the courage to go to the evil gyms, so the evil gyms are now filled with all sorts of people, not all of them are perfect either. If you are terrified of gyms but have never stepped foot in one, maybe now's the time to bust a few more myths?

But if going to the gym, or a Zumba or dance class is too painful we have this amazing thing called the internet. Yes, you can exercise in the comfort, privacy, and security of your own home. You can get dancing or stretching in the living room. You can shut the curtains, no one needs know! There are so many free workouts online - although there are lots of great ones you might also want to pay for. Why not try a free online workout to see if you like it?

I suspect that some people who read this might be convinced to give a virtual class a go, whereas some will still be thinking that attempting a plank, even in the comfort of the lounge is simply never going to happen. And for those people, that's okay too, as long as you find something.

When I was someone who didn't exercise and had no intention of ever really doing so, I found that walking was the way to start moving my body more. I walked a little, then I walked a little more. I walked when previously I'd have driven short distances, I walked up hills and down again. I started small but I felt good about it. I could feel my body moving and even though I wasn't out of breath or sweaty I knew I was beginning to treat myself right.

Nowadays, I still walk, but also, I run. I absolutely know that to any non-runner that will seem unforgivably intimidating. People who run are like people who enjoy long walks, or people who wear lycra to ride a bike. They're aliens - nutters who need their heads examining. I know all this because I wasn't always a runner.

MY RUNNING STORY

I gradually turned into someone who loves walking, and who runs for fun every single day. Slowly. Enjoyably. Let me tell you about the life-changing, life-lengthening running programme called Couch25K that I discovered as an app on my phone (perhaps my husband had rather ambitiously downloaded it) as it certainly wasn't the sort of thing that I'd have been looking to do myself. It is a way of helping couch potatoes (like me, at the time) to run for five kilometres in a relatively short timeframe of just eight weeks. I decided to give it a go - but I believed there was no way on this earth I'd be able to do it. No way!

After a gentle warm-up, the first week kicks off with a 60 second run. It doesn't sound much, but I clearly remember that first 60 seconds, as I was living in Liverpool's Georgian Quarter at the time where the streets weren't very busy. But that didn't make it any less of a shock to the system. In around 2010, this was the first time I had attempted to run in almost two decades. It was hot, hard, and painful. I was very quickly out of breath, in fact, it felt as if my chest was on fire. I counted the seconds down wishing so hard for that first run to end. I was worried that I might have trouble getting home.

I somehow got to the end of the workout which included a few more incredibly short 'runs', and I felt an enormous sense of achievement, like totally enormous. Who would have thought I would get my trainers on and pound the pavements? Since when did I even own any trainers?

Encouraged by my husband and a healthy dose of competitive spirit, I carried on and, we did three of these Couch25K workouts a week. By about Week 4, I was running for five whole minutes at a time, and by Week 5, I was meant to run for 20 minutes. Now, of course, even though I had prepared my body for this through the running I was doing, a whopping 20 minutes seemed so insane that my tiny brain put a stop to it, and I repeated Week 5 at least six times until I went for it, and finally managed to run for 20 minutes.

Don't give up

Now this seems like a stunning success story, doesn't it? There I was, carrying a lot of weight, miserable with myself, but doing something about it, and achieving physical feats I had never thought were possible before. What could possibly go wrong? Back then, and this is a long time ago now, I was fixing my lack of exercise, I was fixing the food I ate, but I had not fixed my brain; I had not fixed how I felt about myself. I did part of

Couch25K. The programme was so amazing it meant that even I, who at the time was at least a size 18 and probably weighed 200 lb could run for 20 minutes. But I didn't carry on. I didn't run for 30 minutes, I never actually ran a 5K, because I just stopped, and I'm not sure why I sabotaged my success like that. It was as if I was shown that anything was possible, but I chose not to take the chance to make the change, to lose weight, and be happy.

There were lots of negative things happening in my life at that point. I had tried to set up a business, but it wasn't working out. A close family member had died. I was struggling financially. I was unhappy with myself. I felt like a failure. I most definitely did not love myself.

If you don't love yourself, it is hard to decide to make lasting changes to your life. You might even find yourself, as I did, making some changes, but the lack of self-love means you'll end up doubting yourself, and failing to follow through. I clearly wanted to be healthier and to lose weight. I plucked up the huge amounts of courage required to start that, I achieved a level of success, but then some nasty part of my brain stopped me from keeping going. My nasty brain still didn't love me enough. I didn't think I deserved to be healthier or slimmer. I thought I had to stay fat and miserable. So, I did, for a little while, at least.

The next time I started Couch25K I was determined to finish it. That was the goal. The goal was to run a 5K. Just one. Years later, and as I was well into my self love journey after I'd had my daughter I decided to run again. I'd been walking more and more intentionally and was losing weight. I started the Couch25K programme again probably when I was a similar weight to the last time, around 200 lb. I started from scratch and found it easy and more enjoyable. I progressed through the weeks, I got to the 20 minute run again, and again I repeated this part several times before progressing. The 8 week programme probably took me 24 weeks and I was fine with that. I did an 'almost 5K' myself and then my friend suggested we do Parkrun. Parkrun is a lot of people running 5K all at once in a park on a Saturday morning and it happens in various locations around the UK. She and I didn't live near each other so we did Parkruns near to our respective houses. I called her afterwards; I was so incredibly overwhelmed by what I'd achieved. Thank you Sara!

Of course if you can run 5K you are generally of the opinion that it's good to do it more than once, so I started running shorter runs regularly and 5Ks once every couple of weeks. Now however, I run every single day. I am currently running 2.5 miles or 4K every day. I ran 5K this morning. It's important to know that not all those annoying people you see running around a park who can do it, were always able to do it. And that even if you aren't one of those annoying people running around a park today, you could be! ;)

ACTIVITY

Activity 9 will help you think deeply about which types of exercise you love, and which types you really don't; and it will help you to get moving with the totally awesome ones.

LOVE MOVING RECAP

Just like with food, it is vital we challenge our beliefs about exercise. I'm living proof that someone who thought exercise was awful and thought I could never run, can turn into a person who looks forward to her runs every day. But starting small and easy is absolutely the right way to go as it's vital that however you move your body, you do it in a way that works for you, that you do it in a way that's enjoyable. I hope you can try out a number of new types of exercise, and I hope you'll find something that sticks.

How to Love Yourself & Lose Weight

The Love Yourself & Lose Weight method is focused on self-love, but there are other important elements to it too. Self-love comes first. Not last. Many people think self-love appears because of weight loss, but it is the other way round. We need to love ourselves first so that we can lose weight. Then of course, we will love ourselves even more!

You may not be feeling the self-love bit yet, but I am going to support you with that. I will help you to understand why self-love is so important, show you how to build it, and then to explain the relationship between self-love and weight loss.

So, do you really need to love yourself to lose weight? Well, yes. And no. Yes, because if you get to the point where you love and respect yourself, you will find it easy and effortless to eat well, exercise (a little) and lose weight healthily. And no, in the sense that as you get to the point where you love and respect yourself, you will probably be eating differently anyway. You will be exercising, and you will be changing your relationship with food.

Love Yourself & Lose Weight is based on the following principles:

- Know your whys - understand why you want to lose weight; delve deep to be clear about why you want this, and why you're deciding to love yourself and to lose weight.

- Love yourself - learn to love yourself more, regardless of what you weigh right now; and really celebrate what makes you uniquely you.

- Eat consciously- Learn to develop new habits that remind you of how great you are every time you eat. Eating is something you are going to be doing a lot of, and it's a good opportunity to continually practise self-love. So, remember to love yourself every time you eat!

- Eat with love - beautiful food helps you to lose weight. When you love yourself, you'll be attracted to beautiful, healthy, happy foods and not the damaging junk that helps you gain weight and makes you miserable.

- Get moving - Loving yourself will make you feel like dancing. Or running, or walking, or like indulging in a spot of shopping, or housework, or whatever floats your boat - regardless, it will make you appreciate your awe-inspiring body (we all have one).

- Share the love - Knowing you love yourself is powerful, and it's kind of contagious too. Tell people that there's something amazing happening over here! Sharing your positivity, ambition and achievements with friends and supporters helps you to stay true to your whys and to feel yet more love from others.

I want to help you to understand and adopt the Love Yourself & Lose Weight method step by step but if you're a super impatient person and you want to do something today to get started, just do these four things:

- Be the good you - Imagine yourself as your fairy godmother or knight in shining armour. You're here to save YOU. Yes, this is exciting because YOU have shown up to save the day, and to rescue yourself from a life of misery, and to deliver yourself into a life of happiness. Get into character. Every time you eat, you need to show up as the capable, wonderful, brave, miracle worker you know you are.

- Be in love with food - Make beautiful food that tastes wonderful and is nutritious. Make the food you'd make for someone you really love. What would you give that person if you had their very best interests at heart and wanted them to live a happy and healthy life? Would it be endless cakes, crisps, chips, chocolate, carbs, and sugar? I doubt it. Think what delicious, fresh, healthy food you'd give to care for and sustain the person you love most in the world. Then make, cook, or order that food.

- Eat with love - Before eating anything drink a glass of water, as it can be easy to mistake thirst for hunger. Drinking water first will also slow you down and remind you to take a moment to think and to remember your whys before launching straight into your food. Think about your weight loss goals and as you eat, savour every mouthful, and eat slowly.

- Stop when full - This is important - many of us don't stop when we're full. We don't stop because we don't notice we're full as we're too busy shovelling food into our mouths. By slowing down your eating, you will notice the feeling of fullness more quickly. As soon as you start to feel full, stop.

These four things feel like second nature to me now, and by doing them, I am losing the weight I want to lose, and it feels easy. By focusing on self-love, beautiful healthy food, and slow conscious eating, I never feel like I am doing without.

Doing all this hasn't always been instinctive for me though. Oh no! I used to turn up as the bad me, the me who didn't give a s*%t if I put on weight, and the me who felt incapable of change. This was the me who didn't appreciate fabulous food, the one who chose cheap empty carbs; the me who felt miserable. I didn't make the choices I'd make for anyone I loved, I basically just treated myself like rubbish. I most definitely did not drink before I ate, nor did I drink much water at all. I ate quickly, I even ate secretly, I ate and ate and ate until I was stuffed. Now I no longer eat like that, and I know I never ever want to go back to my old way of eating. I know I never will.

So being the good you, being in love with food, and eating with love will help you transform your weight, maybe even your life as you start to learn you can achieve your goals. It may not be all that easy at first. You need to practise these new habits, every day, and every time you eat. Perhaps you will feel self-conscious eating super slowly to begin with and that's okay. But actually, eating at a leisurely pace looks a lot less ridiculous than wolfing down your meal in less than two minutes. Try it, then try it again. Keep going, and after a few days you'll find it is enjoyable and exciting to be eating in this way. What have you got to lose?

Love Yourself Every Day

When you love yourself, you will leap out of bed happy each day. Well, you might. Or at least you'll be more likely to leap out of bed happy than if you don't love yourself. I genuinely wake up feeling happy every day as I know I'm achieving my goals and rocking my size 12 outfits, although at the time of writing I have nowhere to wear them due to lockdown.

Leaping out of bed happy is a by-product of self-love and isn't going help you to get self-love in the first place though, so first, we need to look at what we need to do to build the self-love. Remember, self-love is a journey. It's not an on-or-off kind of a thing. You won't just wake up one morning feeling totally in love with yourself. Whilst we all adore a love at first sight story, this is more of a slow burner. And rightly so. We're looking for true love, not just a fling!

What can you do, then, to build self-love? I use a range of techniques; some of them are things you can do once, or once in a while, and others are strategies that you can implement over and over again. Firstly, let's look at some of the stuff you can do every day.

To embed the idea of self-love and to really fall in love with yourself, you're going to have to start first thing in the morning. It is important to wake up well as it sets you up for the whole day and determines how you deal with certain situations. To wake up well you need to have had a good night's sleep, so if you're used to staying up way past your sensible bedtime, you might want to have a think about changing that. Sleep is a healer after all, we need lots of it, not just because we're going to be increasingly active and eating more consciously, but also because we're going to be thinking all these exciting thoughts about how we're amazing; and our subconscious, sleepy brains need time to process that stuff, so it sinks in.

I have read a lot recently about the seemingly bonkers idea of leaping straight out of bed as soon as you wake up. The rationale is that by moving straight away, you simply don't have time for worrying. As someone who definitely does not get straight out of bed when I wake up, I thought I'd try it, albeit reluctantly. I'll be honest, I found it rather hard at first, but then I got a little better at it. I can't claim I leap out of bed straightaway, but I definitely spend less time lying around allowing my brain to wonder and worry. Often, it is better to just get up and get on with it, than it is to lie there thinking about it.

So, get a good night's sleep and get up promptly, and you'll instantly feel more like a go-getter and that anything is possible.

Embrace Affirmations

Your whys and your affirmations are perhaps the most awkward part of this method, especially for those of you who just want to change your eating and exercise regime. Well, this method isn't about just changing your diet or exercise regime, it's about changing you, and how you think about yourself, so you have got to do more than just track your calories and steps each day. You must shape your brain, bust some myths, and reform your beliefs. What has led to so many of us remaining overweight is the idea that we are not worth making the change for. We also tend to believe that this change is incredibly hard or even entirely impossible.

Your affirmations are what will set your brain straight on these matters. You will have written down your affirmations, based on your whys. You need to remember both your affirmations and your whys each day at a specific time to suit you. Pick a quiet time, and just take a minute, sit somewhere quiet and say your whys to yourself in your head, and then, repeat your affirmations. If you want to shout them out loud whilst staring in the bathroom mirror or standing in the middle of your local supermarket, that's fine, but saying them in your head will do.

Every time you eat is a chance to remind your brain that you are an amazing person who is capable of great things, and that you can lose weight, and deserve to do so, or however you want to frame it. I am a firm believer that eating is not just an opportunity to refuel, but it is also a chance to show yourself just how much you care about you. Remember you love yourself. Say it in your head.

Pick one type of exercise you can do each day. This might be walking, or cleaning, and it does not have to involve a trip to a gym. As you move your body, say your affirmations to yourself. By linking your physical activity and your affirmations you are helping your brain to understand that physical activity is going to help you to achieve your goals. You don't need to repeat your affirmations each time you exercise (although I often do), but repeating them as you move your body will help you to remember them and will make it easier for your brain and body to respond to them.

In addition to the strategies that you use every day to build self-love, there's also some fun stuff you can do just once, or once in a while. You will identify and define your whys and write down your affirmations as activities in this book. They're things you do once and use every day. You can of course go back and refine them as they make more and more sense to you and you get to know yourself and your desires better, but they won't change all that much. A more creative, expressive activity perhaps, is to create a vision board.

Make a Vision Board

I bet you know or can guess what this is already. When I first heard about this idea, I thought it was so cringey. Yes, you guessed it, a vision board is basically a board onto which you stick pictures of the things you want. You might put pictures of you when you've lost weight. You might put pictures of your head stuck on someone else's body, or you might put pictures of the clothes you'll wear, the places you'll go and the things you'll see. I got rather creative with mine; it even has a home gym on it!

Vision boards work because they give physical form to an idea. I don't want to sound too mystical at this point, so try to imagine it like this. You've had an idea of yourself being thin. You create a picture of it. You look at the picture of you being thin. Your brain gets the instruction so it can then help you to get what's on the picture. This is not only a fun activity, it's a hugely powerful one. You can put the picture somewhere you'll see it every day. Look at it morning, noon and night if you want to. Look at it when you're eating, when you're making decisions, when you're washing up. The point is, look at it. Let your brain see your desired future reality so it can create it.

ACTIVITY

Perhaps the messiest activity in this book, check out Activity 10 and get creative with a Vision Board.

Love Your Achievements

The Love Yourself & Lose Weight method is fundamentally about love; loving yourself and loving what you are achieving. It is vital you make the time to enjoy your achievements however small they may seem. All your achievements are important, not just reaching a goal weight. By way of an example, here are the things I've achieved and celebrated in the last month.

- I'm going to my best friend's wedding in a couple of weeks and both my options for a wedding guest dress are a size 12. I'm looking forward to being three dress sizes smaller than I was at his last wedding :).

- I bought a pair of zip-up, knee-high boots and didn't have to worry about my calves being too big to do them up.
- As the cold weather's hit, I'm loving wearing my All Saints leather jacket in a size 12. Previously nothing in their stores would go on. Nada, zip.
- I bought running wear from the Nike store. The old me still wonders who this person is!
- I upped my running distance each morning from 1 mile to 1.5 miles, to 2.5 miles which is my new baseline.
- I have lost five pounds in the last month.
- I ran every day for a week.
- I ran every day for six months.
- I feel good about myself when I get dressed.
- I feel good just because.

It is important to reflect occasionally on your accomplishments so that you realise how far you've come. Now I've been doing this a long time, but it is so important to celebrate the achievements you'll make in just the first few days on the Love Yourself & Lose Weight method. For example:

- Celebrate that you're doing this, that you've thought about your whys and written down your affirmations.

- Celebrate the fact that you have decided to love yourself and lose weight. This is huge. It is perhaps the most exciting thing you've done in a long time and will change your life. You've decided. You're committed. This is happening.
- Celebrate that you drank a glass of water before a meal and took a moment to remember you love yourself.
- Celebrate that you thought carefully about a food choice.
- Celebrate that you ate consciously.
- Celebrate that you left some food on your plate.
- Celebrate that you went for a walk or tried some new exercise.
- Celebrate that you love yourself.

Celebrations are important. I don't mean the 'Ooh I've lost two pounds so now I can celebrate with a takeaway' sort of celebrations. No, I mean just taking time to acknowledge your success.

Tracking your achievements is important too, and there are so many ways in which we can track these days. I use Withings Scales which are attached to the HealthMate app. I can track my weight over time. There are charts, graphs and statistics that I could get bothered with if I were that kind of girl, but I just like to use it to know where I am right now. It is good though, seeing just how far I've come. Tracking should not be used in an obsessive way. Don't get weighed every day and get upset about a lack of movement or movement in the wrong direction. Track regularly but periodically so you can see your journey. Tracking helps you to understand when you're likely to hit a goal, and to record when you hit it. But more importantly than just keeping track, use it to celebrate your success, to remind yourself of just how amazing you are.

When to get weighed

So why would you not get weighed every day? Well, our bodies are complex; what shows up on the scales one morning doesn't relate directly to what happened yesterday. Just because you hardly ate much on a Saturday doesn't mean you'll have lost a pound of fat by Sunday. There are lots of reasons why our weight fluctuates as we slim down. Firstly, our bodies take time to process what we eat and the fat we lose. The solids and liquids in our system weigh different amounts day to day. We have hormonal changes (for some of us in a big way). I can gain three pounds in the run up to, and during the first two days of my period, then drop three or even four pounds a day after.

If you get weighed every day, you'll see all this fluctuation. If you're someone who just really wants to know, that's fine, but many of us get put off if we go 'up'. However, it is important to point out that putting on weight does not necessarily mean you have got fatter, but so many people don't realise this. Sure, you might weigh more, but your fat percentage might be down, and your water percentage might be up. Some scales measure all these different changes - but even then, a number that isn't less than the last number can be disheartening.

It isn't essential that you splash out on sophisticated scales that can measure your water and fat content. If you are eating well and exercising, after the first few days when you will lose water, you are guaranteed to start losing fat too.

If you space out your weigh-ins to weekly, you're more likely to drop progressively; each week the scales are more likely to tell you that you weigh less than the last, and you'll feel nothing but positivity. Don't leave it too long though between weigh-ins because they will keep you on track, so you feel accountable.

I am still on the fence, really, when it comes to whether to weigh yourself every day. I used to weigh myself every single day and felt that it helped to remind me of the task ahead. If I had gone up, or not gone down for a while I might be prompted to be more conscious about what I was eating, or to move a little more. For me it was a motivator. Now I weigh myself about once a week, as I prefer the better news I get weekly than the occasionally rather confused news I used to get each morning.

It's up to you, if you're the kind of person who gets really disappointed to the point of giving up, if you go up a pound, do not get weighed every day. If you want to know and learn from the granular data and are okay with the fluctuations, then go for the daily update.

ACTIVITY

Get tracking with Activity 11. It's fun and easy - and puts you in control.

What it takes to lose just one pound of fat

When someone starts a weight loss plan and is super happy on day two as they have lost a couple of pounds, I feel a bit awkward, because the truth is they have probably just lost water. It takes quite a bit of effort to shift 2 pounds of fat.

Now, I know you understand this stuff, but I want to remind you that a pound of fat equates to 3,500 calories. That is to say that to lose a pound of fat you need to burn 3,500 calories more than you eat. Unless you exercise like crazy, you're unlikely to burn 3500 calories in one day, let alone burn 3,500 calories on top of what you eat. Let's say you normally eat and burn 2,000 calories to stay the same weight. Now let's imagine you eat 1,750 calories and burn off 250 calories through exercise; you will have created a calorie deficit of 500 calories. At this rate it will take a whole week to have burned off an extra 3500 calories - to lose one pound of fat. You could eat fewer calories and do more exercise and your daily deficit will go up. Let's imagine you eat 1,250 calories a day (you'll be hungry), and you burn 250 calories a day through exercise on top of your normal activity, you'd have a deficit of 1,000 calories.

1000 x 7 = 7000. That's two pounds of fat that it's possible to lose in a week.

Don't get overexcited at the start

If you start a diet on one day and eat half the food you usually eat (which often happens on diets as they are restrictive), your body will be lighter the next day simply because it has less stuff in it. You are emptying your stomach and intestines so you will be lighter. In the next few days of any diet or weight loss method, you will lose more pounds. As your body has less food in it, you will also lose water. Certain diets also accelerate water loss early on.

The early effects of dieting mean you lose weight, but not necessarily fat. People often feel excited at this point, as they see the pounds dropping off, assuming it's all fat loss, which it isn't. Following this honeymoon period of rapid weight loss, it can be disheartening as the progress slows. It is hugely important to celebrate your early achievements, but you need to understand what your achievements are. Don't celebrate that you are able to lose five pounds of fat a week if you've lost five pounds of water and stomach contents. Do celebrate that you've made a decision to make a change in your life, and that you're on your journey. Do expect that you will drop some weight quickly but understand that processing and losing fat weight might take a little longer. Be okay with that. This is a process not a quick fit. In the next few weeks, your weight loss will slow down, and you will start to understand how long it takes for your body to lose fat. Understand it, don't force it; listen to your body, work with it.

Losing two pounds of fat per week is considered quick. Losing one pound per week is a sensible pace. Now, we're all keen to get on with it when we start, but as you get into it, you need your weight loss to be sustainable. If whatever you're doing to lose wight leaves you feeling weak and unnourished you simply won't be able to stick at it. Many people achieve a rapid drop at first, then see their weight loss slowing. It's so important to celebrate success that isn't just about weight loss. Ultimately, losing a lot of weight takes a long time; it just does, and it's important to go into it expecting that. There's no quick fix that works; we need true lasting change here. Things that are worth doing are worth doing well.

After the initial body shock and weight drop, your real weight loss starts. Your body will settle into a rhythm and routine. Your brain needs to settle in with it too. No one can know how quickly you will lose weight. You can attempt to make it quicker, but whatever you do, it must be sustainable. The best way to think about this is to treat it as an experiment. As you settle into your new routine, learn from your body. Learn what it needs and wants, learn the pace at which your body can process fat whilst keeping you feeling sated and happy.

And remember, any thoughts that things are not happening quickly enough are not really very helpful to you. If you feel impatient then you're not appreciating the wonderful stuff that's happening. Remember, you've made an amazing decision, you're learning to love yourself, you're making changes; your body will respond.

HELP WITH SELF-IMPROVEMENT

This self-love and weight loss journey is indeed one of self-improvement. You will improve your mind and body AND outlook on life, indeed everything. I hope it will be transformational and inspirational. I hope and believe you will enjoy it, but loving yourself doesn't have to mean you can't get help when you need it. It doesn't mean you have to be a martyr!

We all occasionally need external inputs to help us feel amazing on the inside and sometimes it's fair to say we need a little pampering. Looking back at my Instagram posts these last few months, there were a lot of trips to the hair salon; it seems hair and nails have been a big part of my journey. I managed to go to the sunbed shop and the hair salon a lot, all while adhering to the lockdown restrictions, of course. It's fair to say that my beauty treatments became part and parcel of my self-love routine. As they should. After all, you don't want to be someone who loses weight but fails to buy any new clothes or who doesn't bother to get great hair to match your fantastic body.

Pampering by way of beauty treatments is essential for those of us who have self-love. You need to tell yourself you're worth it. Get your hair and nails done.

Get a tan, get your brows done, or whatever floats your boat.

For most of us, this is about as far as we go with pampering treatments. But some of us take it further. Just as I've discussed that you have to love yourself BEFORE you can lose weight, you also have to love yourself BEFORE you can give yourself the permission, or impetus to go out and get pampered. You could imagine that you might love yourself more after getting your hair done or after sorting your eyebrows out. But this is not the case. The self-love must come first to enable you to do the self-care.

Look good, feel good

I want to explain that in addition to your new self-love and weight loss activities, it's okay to get a little extra help to feel amazing and it's okay to use your newfound self-love to fix, well whatever you like. Also, losing weight can radically transform how people look, but there are some things that can't be addressed by diet or exercise.

There's also no judgement here about surgery. I shouldn't really have to say that, because as an advocate for self-love that 'no judgement' thing should be obvious. But just to be clear, surgery, like anything else is a personal choice, and is no way at odds with self-love. Loving yourself does not mean you can't have surgery, just as having surgery doesn't mean you'll automatically love yourself. Your newfound self-love may well encourage you to make other changes in your life. The self-love movement empowers people to love and care for themselves, to feel loved and special and capable of great things. I have felt that power, I've felt accepting of my body and I've desired change.

But self-love doesn't mean that you can't have surgery to further improve yourself, it doesn't mean that surgery is somehow cheating or a shortcut. Far from it. I see a lot of people who have lost masses of weight. After substantial weight loss, unfortunately, our bodies don't automatically spring back to how they were before we put on weight. Generally, people who have lost lots of weight will carry loose skin. This isn't something that can be improved or removed through diet or exercise. For many people in that situation, they choose surgery to remove the loose skin and to help them feel fully happy with themselves. I think that's awesome.

The surgical route

I also see a lot of people online who've had surgery to lose weight. Bariatric or 'weight loss' surgery helps so many. Whilst it wasn't my route, although I did consider it, I don't think this is in any way an easy option. Don't think that just because someone is having bariatric surgery, that they can get by without loving themselves. No, I think the contrary is true. You need to love yourself to go ahead with any surgery, you need to love yourself to learn how to eat and exercise well, you need to love yourself to feel great now and into the future.

I read a lot about people who had bariatric surgery but weren't mentally prepared for what was to come next - weight loss, changing shape, not being physically able to eat how they ate before. Self-love is absolutely required by anyone embarking on a massive change. You have to love yourself before and during the change, not just afterwards.

My surgery story

As someone who has been much larger, after I lost weight, I suffered from having loose skin in places that simply wouldn't shift through diet and exercise. I felt this was entirely unfair, I had achieved so much in losing weight but had issues that basically I couldn't do anything about. While I don't strive for perfect, I absolutely strive to have a body I am proud of. I am not someone who'd ever thought I'd have plastic surgery. But this wasn't just about a little improvement here or there, nor was it about fitting an ideal or stereotype; for me, this was a big deal as I felt I had a big problem.

In December 2020, five years after I originally lost 85 pounds, I decided to have brachioplasty (that's arm lift surgery), as there was simply no way I was going to have arms that fitted with the rest of me without surgery. Now at 45, I am now pretty happy with my 'normal' size 12 body. And by 'normal' I mean lumpy and bumpy and absolutely perfectly imperfect.

I had surgery to help finish up my transformation and I am so overwhelmingly pleased that I did. Of course, surgery is expensive and I am incredibly lucky that it was something I was able to do. I worked super hard and saved for a long time to be able to do it, by the way. I am sharing this with you because it's important to understand that self-love enabled me to work hard, to save the money, to lose the weight, to get ready for surgery, to heal afterwards and so on. Self love helped me make a change in my life. Self love is not however, the result of surgery.

We all need a little help wherever we are on our self-love journey. We all absolutely need pampering. And if we need to make some bigger changes, then that is fine too as long as we love ourselves first and are doing it for the right reasons. It's also really important to remember there's no such thing as perfect. I, for one am not working towards a perfect body, but I am working towards a happy version of me. We're all different, so we all need to find out own version of ourselves we're happy with. And we're all a work in progress, I most certainly am - and that's ok. It's ok to be on the journey - now let's enjoy it!

SETTLE IN FOR THE JOURNEY

The start is perhaps the hardest part, and it is the part you really do have to get right. It's not about waking up one day and suddenly being the kind of person who eats super healthily, who works out, or who can say no to wine when out with your friends. Especially if this isn't who you've been so far. And if you haven't been this 'amazing' person, and if you haven't done any of these things, it's unlikely that you'll be able to suddenly leave a bunch of old habits behind just like that. This would be a massive ask. Massive! It is, however, something that some people can do, but they are few and far between, and most of us who attempt this fail at it after a few weeks because it's just not sustainable.

No, the start is not about some mad body shock, bootcamp or enduring exercise regime with a personal trainer at dawn every day. If this was what it took, then hardly anyone would reach the finish line. The assumption that we need to suddenly become someone else, overnight, is a problem in itself. The idea that once we've magically become someone else in our sleep, that we'll be cured of our old habits, and will have become a super achiever is not realistic or appealing, frankly. The problem with this idea is that it fails to recognise that in our current 'before' state, we are capable of great things.

We must not wait for that long-awaited magic day when we will suddenly see everything differently. Why not? Because that day could be any day. That day could be today. And that person who is capable of great achievements IS NOT another person, another version of you that you've not yet met. That person, who is capable of great things is YOU!

Waiting for some magic day, waiting for you to mysteriously turn into someone else, waiting for you to be suddenly capable of eating a totally healthy diet and working out every day, is silly. That day never comes for most of us, so we just feel let down when our future magic selves never show up.

But with our growing self-love we really are capable of great things, of radical change. Whoever we are today, we can show up. We the imperfect, underachievers in the weight loss department, we who have put weight on, we who have not exercised (much), we who have overeaten, we who are fed up with this, we who know we deserve better, we who are starting to love ourselves - we can absolutely show up and make a start.

The people who can show up and make a change are the ones who have decided. In fact, the decision is the start; once you have decided, you're already on your journey.

FORGET WILLPOWER

If you are losing weight through willpower or denying yourself the ability to eat food you think you love, then yeah, you can 'stick to it' when everything goes your way but any spanner in the works will put you off track. I talked earlier about willpower and why it's not necessary; in fact, it's unhelpful. If you feel you need to summon all the willpower in the world to do something unpleasant, you may do it for a bit, but you won't continue long- term, no matter what it is.

But if you learn to love yourself, you are losing weight by positively choosing to eat beautiful food and you're enjoying eating beautiful food and enjoying losing weight. A setback for someone who is enjoying a new way of eating is unlikely to stop them wanting to eat beautiful food. Once you start to enjoy moving your body through positive exercise, nothing is going to get in the way.

Often, we associate 'bad foods', usually carbs and sugar, with comfort eating. Pizza, ice cream, and chocolate are the things we turn to in a crisis or when we need cheering up. This is fuelled by messages from the media and the advertising industry; we're all familiar with their narratives. If you still believe that empty carbs are in some way pleasurable, you may turn to them for comfort. But if you learn to see empty fat-creating carbs for what they are, then you will no longer crave them in the same way - even when life presents you with challenges. In fact, as someone who loves yourself, eats beautifully, and enjoys losing weight, the idea of stuffing your face with chocolate might smack of self-harm and isn't something you'd want to do to yourself.

So, I'll say it again - forget willpower. It's important to remember the idea that you don't want to eat foods that do you no good. Instead, you want to eat foods that make you feel special and loved, and you want to enjoy eating beautifully.

BE PATIENT

I've talked about how losing two pounds a week is quick but losing one pound a week is great. To some people, me included at one point, that sounds like terribly slow progress. I get it – you don't want to wait for 50 weeks to lose 50 pounds, right? Well, if you did lose 50 or even 100 pounds and it took you a year that would still be amazing, wouldn't it? Especially as your love for yourself will grow every day.

Weight loss is a journey, it's not an event. That's why so many people fail at it; because they think it is a quick process that will soon be over – and then they can start eating as they did before. This is why so many people opt for restrictive diets that are sold as a quick fix, and they expect to lose all their weight in a matter of weeks, or a few months at least. Perhaps they do lose a lot of weight, but they then stop the diet and put all the weight back on.

It doesn't really matter how long it takes to lose weight, as long as you're learning to love yourself and moving towards your desired goal. You must be committed to the journey. And while you might see rapid results, you may have times when your progress seems slower but remember that speed isn't important. If you take self-love with you on your journey, the journey will be enjoyable.

This is a journey not an event

The Love Yourself and Lose Weight method is less like a prescriptive daily regime and more like a set of principles to live by for as long as you like, but most likely forever.

Who wouldn't want to love themselves forevermore? Who would want to learn to love themselves for a period of time, lose weight, then stop loving themselves? No one, I guess.

Self-love is something you will build from day one, from the decision point. It will build and grow until it becomes second nature. The best bit is that it should stay with you forever. This method is about learning to love yourself, losing weight and feeling happy to be you. It isn't instant, although some changes will be quick. The process of change is a long one, some changes will happen today, some this week, some in a few months and some later on. And that's okay. Your mind is changing. Your body is changing. You are changing. Sometimes your body changes, and your mind needs time to catch up; sometimes your mind changes and your body needs time to catchup. This is all okay. Just know that this is a journey.

Quick fixes are temporary if they work at all. If you're substantially 'overweight' right now and have been for a while and want not to be ever again, then any method that is temporary simply won't serve you well in the long-term. If you focus on diet alone and don't think about changing how you feel about yourself, there'll be no way your brain can keep up with the weight loss. If your brain is still in weight gain mode, it will have a very hard time helping you to maintain your healthy weight when you've lost some. To lose weight and to keep it off, you need to make permanent lifelong changes. Or rather as you evolve, and your sense of self-love develops, your mind will adapt and will keep finding new ways to help you stay on the right track and to enjoy your new healthy body.

ACTIVITY

Activity 12 helps you to think about why you really don't need willpower because you really don't love bad foods all that much.

Lifelong change cannot be achieved in an instant. It takes time. It takes practice. It requires you to grow mentally along the journey. It needs you to realise that this is a journey, and to be prepared and happy to make a start, not knowing exactly how you'll get to your destination, but that you will get there. And once you're there, self-love will help you to stay there.

Undoing the years of not loving yourself is easy

I regret spending too many years not loving myself. My lack of self-love was just so obvious for everyone to see. When I look back at pictures of myself in my early thirties, I don't really recognise myself. For starters, I now look nothing like I did then. I look younger at 45 than I did at 33. I am considerably smaller, massively fitter, and insanely happier. The lack of self-love in my early thirties led me to gain weight, to not really develop my career properly, and to lower my ambitions, in well, pretty much every area of my life.

Years went by before I finally got it. I initially thought that it would take me a very long time to reverse all those years of not loving myself, but I was wrong. If you're feeling that because you've spent a long time out of love with yourself, that this is going to be a long slog, don't! The brilliance of self-love is that once you start to get it, it snowballs. Just like falling in love with someone else, you'll fall in love with you. Self-love builds quickly, then that's just the way you are.

Of course, losing large amounts of weight does take time but the self-love bit can be super speedy. And once you get it, you'll never look back and you'll find your weight loss goals easy to achieve.

ACTIVITY

Visualising progress on a timeline can be extremely helpful as it shows how one great thing leads to another. Take a look at Activity 13 and get planning.

FALLING OFF THE HORSE

Are you raring to go right now? Do you feel super positive and like nothing can stop you? I don't want to stop you, of course I want you to be raring to go, to be planning your grocery shopping and thinking about how awesome you're going to look and feel when you've lost weight. I encourage you; do start now. Start right away.

But be warned and expect that at some point you will fall off the horse you're about to get on. I don't know anyone who, after years of treating themselves badly, has started a weight loss journey and never looked back. I don't know anyone who's never found it hard, faltered, or fallen off that horse completely. To start something, succeed, and never fall off, would be rare if not impossible.

But why do we fall off the proverbial horse if this, or any other weight loss method works so well? That is a good question, and one I've asked myself time and time again as I've flailed around eating a secret stash of chocolate after secret stash of chocolate. Why, oh why on earth, after losing over 80 pounds, would I suddenly stop losing weight, stop treating myself well, start treating myself badly, and making myself feel utterly miserable? But perhaps the question I should have asked is why did I stop loving myself?

Self-sabotage is one reason. The idea that as we reach our goal we panic and question subconsciously whether we really want to make substantial changes. Our brains work in mysterious, and occasionally, terrible ways. Maybe for you it's not about self-sabotage. For you, there might be other factors at play; events that you just can't deal with or physical issues - perhaps an injury. Or perhaps you've just become too comfortable with your current self.

Whatever the reason, most people fall off the horse at some point for some reason. And as we fall off, we forget to love ourselves, we forget our whys, we stop saying our affirmations and then we start with the bad habits again. The good news is that this happens to the best of us. Yes, even after losing over 80 pounds. (Are you freaking kidding me?)

Falling off sucks big time. Even in the first day or so you know it sucks. Many of us who fall off the horse pretend it doesn't suck, at least at first. There'll be some things you pretend you're enjoying about having lost your way. You tell yourself all sorts of nonsense about how much you're enjoying eating chocolate and chips. You may even really try to enjoy the ice cream binge but deep down you'll be feeling the pain. The crappy, sucky pain of the knowledge that you're not bringing your good you to the dinner table. The sense of disappointment that your fairy godmother has failed to show up and that the only person you can turn to for help is bad you.

If (and I do mean when) I fall off my horse and languish in a chocolate mess for a few days, I feel like utter crap. Falling off the horse is not a lavish, hedonistic frenzy of beautiful food and relaxation. It's not about overindulging in a divinely sophisticated patisserie or developing an interest in exotic French cheeses. Oh no, for me, falling off the horse involves large quantities of bad, cheap food, made mainly from sugar. I tend to overeat food I know makes me feel rubbish then I wonder why I feel so bad. Then I beat myself up emotionally, then I eat more chocolate, or ice cream. Then I feel doubly bad and so it all continues. The emotional battle in my brain wages on and I feel powerless to stop it.

It bloody sucks. This happens to most of us. Sadly, this, or something like this, will probably happen to you.

Please don't feel at this stage that there's no point in embarking on your journey if you're only going to fall off the horse at some point. I have good news for you: getting back on is easy.

When people embark on a restrictive diet and then fail to keep it up, the horse is harder to get back on. If you lose weight through self-love and you fall off, it's not a diet you're stopping or failing at, it's just a blip, an interruption to your good feelings and sense of self-love. The great news is that loving yourself is something that's always easy to get back. With self-love, it's easy to get right back on your horse and to ride off into your sunset.

So why do we lose our sense of self-love at all if it's so powerful? Well, I'm not perfect, you're not perfect, indeed no one is perfect. We're all on a journey, and on any journey, you occasionally slow down a little, get stuck somewhere for a while or take a wrong turn. And like any journey, when any of those things happen, you eventually find the resources you need to get back on your way.

As I have said, if you love yourself enough, then getting back on that proverbial horse won't be too difficult, but it's important, nevertheless, to take your 'fall' seriously. If you have spent a few days or weeks (or months) forgetting to love yourself, then you need a reset. You need to go deep and think carefully about what you want and how awesome and capable you are.

When I forget myself and I forget to love myself, and I end up overeating for a while, I know it's important that I pick myself up quickly. To do this, I go back to the beginning, and I revisit my whys, and make sure they're still applicable. Then I decide to commit to losing weight all over again. Perhaps I decided to lose a certain amount of weight and I achieved that, and my decision is now out of date. A new decision is always an excellent catalyst for me; the act of deciding again instills self-love, and always ensures I am back on track. If you do find yourself falling off the horse, follow the simple steps again and commit to loving yourself and you will easily get back on your way too.

SHARING THE LOVE

As you get into your stride with this and see the pounds dropping off there will be huge cause for celebration. What a great feeling that is! Loving your achievements can be done alone, but it can be done with others too. You might feel that the world isn't ready for your weight loss success, or that you aren't ready to share with your loved ones what you have decided to do in case they're not supportive. Those closest to us aren't always the best people to share this stuff with for lots of reasons, so it's totally okay if you don't want to share it with them. It's also okay if you want to wait a while to start sharing, to make sure you're on track and that this isn't some fad diet or quick fix. (It isn't!)

Lots of people turn to social media to share their story as it's not only a great way to help you celebrate, as others will celebrate with you, but it's also an effective means of holding yourself accountable. If you post that you're going to walk 10,000 steps to all your friends on Facebook, then you'd better well walk 10,000 steps. If you post pictures of your dinner on Instagram with the hashtag #eatbeautifully #consciouseating and #loveyourselfandloseweight you're less likely to wolf down the dinner, then eat a double helping of choc-chip ice cream for pudding.

Sharing your story on social media isn't for everyone, and you need to find the channel that works for you. For me, whilst Facebook is for staying in touch with friends on more general topics, Instagram is a lively, supportive community of people interested in self-love and weight loss - and a perfect space to share my self-love journey. If you do take to Instagram, there'll be others there too, and it's a great way to find out what they're up to and to support and learn from each other.

ACTIVITY

Activity 14 is all about sharing. You can go big or go small, but spreading the love is always good.

LOVE YOURSELF & LOSE WEIGHT RECAP

I hope you've enjoyed learning about how to love yourself. It still seems silly that we need to learn to love ourselves, but sadly, many of us do. But once we do, anything is possible; we become superhuman versions of ourselves, capable of great things.

In this section we've covered the fundamentals of the LYALW method, of settling in for the journey and considering this to be a process: a journey and not an event. It's vital to have a sense of realism, to abandon perfectionism and to accept and love yourself, celebrating all your wonderful achievements.

For me, building self love has meant I'm able to share my story with others, to help others to love themselves. Will you share your story too?

Your

Success Story

Many of us wait years or decades even before we make the weight loss changes that we know we want and need to make. We wait a long time for many reasons. Fear is one of them; we feel afraid we might fail, and in some cases, that we might succeed. I know that sounds strange but if you have been big for a long time, then losing weight can be an incredible adjustment to make.

I hope that reading this book has made you feel less afraid, as you now know all the reasons why people fail to lose weight. You also know that this method isn't a quick fix or hard to follow. It works; it worked for me, and it can work for you too.

But having discussed the theory, and my tips for success, the following section of this book is all about you. I've created a few simple, and hopefully, enjoyable activities to get you started, that should help you to stay on the right track for the first 12 months. This is your self-love toolkit, and self-love journal.

You can complete the activities as you read the book, or all at once at the end, or you can keep dipping in and out. It's entirely up to you. Here are the things you need to do to get started:

- Know your whys.
- Create your affirmation.
- Say your affirmation.
- Define your decision.
- Say your decision.
- Eat consciously.
- Eat happy foods.
- Get moving.
- Create your vision.
- Get tracking.
- Forget willpower.
- Plan your journey.
- Share your success.

MY SUCCESS STORY

This is my self-love and weight loss journal.

My name is...

Today's date is...

Before starting this, I love myself ....%.

I'd like to love myself ....%.

My starting weight is ....

My goal weight is...

My whys are:

....

....

....

....

My BHAGs (Beautiful Happy Awesome Goals) are:

....

....

....

....

My daily affirmation is:

....

....

....

....

ACTIVITY 1: KNOW YOUR WHYS

1. Write your whys in the space below. Write lots of them. See this as an 'ideas' session. Think of as many whys as you can. It doesn't matter if they're any good, or the right ones for now. Just get them down.

2. Circle the ones that make the most sense for you.
Do not feel guilty about not writing whys for other people (like 'I want to be able to run long distances for my dog') just write whys for YOU.

My whys #1

....

....

....

....

....

....

....

3. Now cross out any whys that are about removing a negative thing, for example, 'I don't want to be unable to buy clothes in regular stores,' or 'I don't want to miss out on sunbathing on a fancy yacht in the Caribbean.'

4. Rewrite them below as a 'positives' such as, 'I want to buy skimpy beach dresses and feel great in them.' or 'I want to feel fabulous lounging around on a yacht.'

My whys #2

....

....

....

....

....

....

....

Circle three to five whys for your shortlist.

5. Write out your top three whys neatly with pride. Add some sparkle if you wish!

My whys #3

....

....

....

....

....

....

....

....

....

....

....

You've done brilliantly if you can do this already. It took me many months to fully define my whys. And I review and renew them often. This will probably still be a work in progress, and we'll come back to these later, but for now you have your whys. This is amazing. You're amazing!

ACTIVITY 2: CREATE AN AFFIRMATION

1. Think about what you'd like your brain to know (to really know) about the fact that you love yourself or are starting to love yourself.

2. Write at least two of these things below or make up your own:

I <heart> me.
I love me.
I love myself.
I'm worthy of love.

....

....

....

....

3. Now think about why you're so awesome, focus on your special skills, the amazing stuff you've done and so on.

4. Write at least two of these things or make up your own.

I'm capable of achieving my goals.
I'm freaking awesome.
I'm amazing / wonderful / gorgeous.
I'm kind / generous / giving.
I bring joy / fun / help /creativity /glamour, whatever it is you bring, to the party.

....

....

....

....

5. Now think about how deserving you are. We often feel undeserving of moving forward or making a change, so it's vital you consider just how absolutely deserving you are of what you want to achieve. You deserve this!

6. Write at least two of these things below or make up your own. Make sure you focus on the fact that you deserve what you desire.

I deserve to lose weight / to be thin.

I deserve to wear pretty / fabulous clothes.
I deserve to be a healthy weight.

. . . .

. . . .

. . . .

. . . .

7. Circle one affirmation from each section. Rewrite the circled affirmation from each section to create a three-part affirmation. You'll start to use this affirmation today and you'll use it several times each day until you truly believe it.

For example:
I love me.
I'm awesome.
I deserve to reach and to maintain a healthy weight.

Your 3 part affirmation

. . . .

. . . .

. . . .

ACTIVITY 3: SAY YOUR AFFIRMATION

Ready to start saying your affirmation out loud?

Good.

So here we go. Find somewhere private and quiet. Preferably with a mirror, although you don't have to say it in the mirror if you don't want to.

Get ready then simply say the words out loud.

There, that wasn't so hard, was it?

Does it feel good? Does it feel awkward? Do you believe you? How much do you believe you?

Notice how this feels. It's totally okay if this feels weird. It's also totally okay if you totally believe what you are telling yourself - this is what we want, this is where we are headed. Wherever you are on the scale of 'this is weird' to 'this is awesome,' that's fine. As I said, practice makes perfect, and in a short time, this will be something you look forward to. I promise.

Now say them again and then commit to saying them to yourself several times a day.

If you're looking for an easy way to remember to say them to yourself, you can repeat them every time you eat. In fact, saying your affirmations before you eat, slows you down and enables you to eat consciously.

ACTIVITY 4: DEFINE YOUR DECISION

So now we're going to define your decision. After all, you can't make a decision unless you're 100% clear about what it is.

Here are some suggestions for how to define a decision:

I have decided to love myself and lose weight.
I have decided to love myself and lose 10 pounds.
I have decided to love myself and lose 20 pounds.
I have decided to love myself and be a size 10.
I have decided to love myself and reach and maintain a healthy weight.

You can add a bit of your own personal desires here if you like: 'I have decided to love myself, lose 40 pounds and look and feel great in hot pants and cowboy boots.'

The more specific the better. It's always better to put a measurable goal in your mind so your brain knows exactly what it needs to do to help you.

1. Write down your decision.

....

. . . .

. . . .

. . . .

. . . .

2. Can you finesse it at all? Are you 100% happy with it? Is it specific enough? Is it measurable?

3. Now complete the decision details on the next page. The next page allows you to define your decision, when you'll make the decision, and why.

You'll create something like this:

On Saturday, 3rd October, I am making a decision to lose 40 pounds and to feel happy and healthy because I want to live a long, healthy, happy life with my family. I'm doing this because I love myself. I'm amazing and I deserve to be a healthy weight and feel great.

MY DECISION

On ....(today's date)

I'm making the decision to:

....

....

....

....

I'm doing this because:

....

....

....

ACTIVITY 5: MAKE YOUR DECISION

Okay so now you've defined your decision, you can make the decision.

Skip this bit at your peril - the act of making the decision is incredibly important.

1. Consider when works for you.

2. Consider where works for you.

3. Know that this is happening; have certainty that once decided, it will happen.

4. Make your decision.

ACTIVITY 6: DEFINE YOUR GOALS

Now it's time to define your BHAGs. Remember that's Beautiful, Happy, Awesome Goals. This should be fun.

1. Write down one amazing thing that you did. If you need inspiration, how about winning the three-legged race at sports day, a pub quiz or a baking competition – anything!

. . . .

2. Write down one amazing thing you did for someone else. We can't all be life-saving medics, but there's a good chance that you've helped someone with something along the way.

. . . .

3. Write down something awesome that you'd like to do for someone you love. Maybe you'd like to take a relative somewhere amazing or teach someone how to play the guitar.

. . . .

4. Now write down something you'd like to do for yourself.

. . . .

. . . .

. . . .

5. Recognise that you're capable of many beautiful things. Sometimes you are capable of awesome things. You're capable of creating joy and happiness.

The rules for creating your BHAGs

Your goals are different from your decision. Your decision just states that you have decided to make a change. Whereas the goals are things that you will achieve along the journey. Some goals will be weight-related, some will not. Remember we are trying to create BHAGs: Beautiful, Happy, Awesome goals.

Beautiful - It must come from a position of love, and it must be something that you want to do for yourself as someone you really love, and think is amazing.

Happy - It must make you feel happy. This can't be something you will worry that you can't achieve. It can't be fragile. And it can't be something you won't tell anyone just in case. It must be awesome – that's all.

Now write down three goals.

1..

2..

3..

ACTIVITY 7: EAT CONSCIOUSLY

I want you to remember how to make positive choices around food - conscious choices. Before eating, buying, or ordering anything to eat, you should ask yourself the questions below. You can tear out the next page of the book and stick it on your fridge or wherever you'll see it most, so that you have a reminder.

1. Next time you eat, ask yourself these questions:

Is this what I really want?
Do I want this because I've just seen an advert for it?
Why do I want this?
Is this going to sustain me?
Is this going to make me feel great?
How amazing is this going to make me feel?
Is this what I'd choose for the person I love most in the world?

2. Practise asking yourself these questions every time you eat.

3. As you're making decisions about ordering, buying, or preparing, any food, get into the habit of asking yourself these questions.

JUST CHECKING...

Cut this out as a handy checklist to keep by the fridge / on your desk / wherever.

Is this food what I really want to eat?

Why do I want this food?

Do I want this because I've seen an ad for it?

Is this food going to sustain me?

Is this food going to make me feel great?

How amazing is this going to make me feel?

Is this the food I would choose for the person I love most in the world?

ACTIVITY 8: EAT HAPPY FOODS

Now it's time to really get to know your happy foods. It's likely that what you previously thought of as your happy foods aren't going to be your happy foods for much longer. To really help you think about happy (and miserable) foods, it's helpful to write some lists.

Over time, this list may change, and some foods may even swap lists. That's okay. We're all learning and evolving.

1. Write a list of foods that make you happy here.

. . . .

. . . .

2. Write a list of foods that make you feel unhappy.

. . . .

. . . .

3. Just have a think about that. Are you sure the foods are in the right list? Do they make you happy? It's okay to move some of them around.

ACTIVITY 9: CREATE YOUR VISION

This is a superb activity for anyone to do at practically any time, for any reason whatsoever. It's fun, inspirational, and helps stretch your imagination.

1. Get a piece of cardboard or a fancy pin-board of a reasonable size.

2. Find pictures of how you want to look, and include the clothes, jewellery, and adornments you want to wear, and then add things you want to be doing, and the places you want to go when you've lost weight.

3. Find pictures of other things that represent how your life will be when you've achieved your goals. This might be where you'll live, where you'll visit on holiday, who you'll be with. Find amazing things you want in your future.

4. Print them out.

5. Cut them out.

6. Stick them together on the board to make a fancy montage of your future reality.

7. Proudly display your vision board where you can see it every day.

8. Take a good long look at it every day. Feel excited. You can make it happen.

ACTIVITY 10: GET MOVING

People who exercise don't necessarily love all forms of exercise. I love running and I would quite like swimming if I could be bothered with soggy changing rooms, but I ain't ever gonna be playing football or rugby or hockey. I am not a team sports kinda girl and I find the hassle of driving to classes annoying but I love a bit of yoga in the comfort and privacy of my living room.

This activity is about getting you to think about what exercise you like and what you don't like. It's about helping you to understand that doing a bit of relaxed yoga at home is amazingly good for you and that you don't need to go out and join the local rugby team. On the other hand, if you want to go and join the bootcamp in your local park and have a muddy, angry instructor shout at you at 9am on a Saturday, you can do that too. If that's what floats your boat.

1. Write down six types of exercise you have never done or never want to do.

....
....
....
....
....
....
....

2. Write down six types of exercise you think you could have a go at. Yep, six. (Don't worry, you don't need to do all six.)

....
....
....
....
....
....
....

3. Write down one type of exercise you really want to have a go at from the top six.

....

4. Write down one physical activity you're going to do today. (This is really happening). Eeek!

....

5. Write down one type of exercise you haven't done before that you're going to try this week.

....

6. Open your calendar or diary and schedule in the thing you're going to try for the first time.

7. Write down what time you're going to do some physical activity today.

8. Do it!

ACTIVITY 11: GET TRACKING

Find a way to track your activity. I am lucky enough to have been given an Apple Watch for my birthday, so I use that, and I love it. Other fitness tackers will do a great job too. This is about you simply knowing what's what and getting a fuzzy feeling as you see your activity levels increase over time. While some fancy fitness trackers may cost a tidy sum, there are plenty out there that will do the basics of tracking your steps without breaking the bank.

If you ain't loving the idea of wearable technology that's fine. You can write down your activities on paper. That's all good too. It's just about knowing and keeping track.

1. Get a tracker and use it for a week.

2. Armed with knowledge about your current activity levels, fill this in.

Before starting this method, my daily exercise includes:

....

My daily step count is usually...............................

I will increase this to.....................................

I think this will make me feel absolutely

....

ACTIVITY 12: FORGET WILLPOWER

I have written about why willpower is not a helpful thing, or something you need when you love yourself and lose weight. I want to make sure that you understand this, so this activity is here just to reinforce why you won't be needing willpower at all.

1. Write a list of foods that have made you put weight on:

....

....

....

....

....

....

....

....

2. Think about how eating those foods made you feel. Write how eating these foods really made you feel:

....

....

....

....

....

....

....

....

3. Now write how attracted you are to these foods:

....

....

....

....

You might start this exercise assuming you love pizza or chocolate, but when you think carefully, the words you write to describe how eating them makes you feel are not words like 'energised', 'nourished', 'cared for'. No, they're words like 'stuffed', 'bloated' and 'harmed'.

When you start to understand this, and as you understand this more and more each day, you can forget willpower and learn to love what you eat as you love yourself.

ACTIVITY 13: PLAN YOUR JOURNEY

This activity will help you to plan your journey. We're going to use this to help you think about the future, and to get you really excited about your long-term goal as well as the journey to get there.

IN FIVE YEARS' TIME

....

IN THREE YEARS' TIME

....

IN ONE YEAR'S TIME

....

IN SIX MONTHS' TIME

....

TODAY

....

1. First write your start point under 'Today'.

2. Then write your one or three year destination. This could be something like: 'I want to weigh 10 stones,' or 'my aim is to have a BMI of 23.' This is a long way away from today. That may seem scary, but don't let it put you off.

3. Then think a couple of years from the point at which you reach your destination. You want to be one of those 'amazing' people, who keep their weight off years later don't you? So, pick something to put in the five years away space.

4. Now go back and add some other nice things you'd like to do for yourself along your journey. I have added all sorts of lovely stuff in mine like how I want to go on holiday and feel great in a swimsuit, how I want to enjoy sending time with my daughter, that I want to run longer distances and get fitter, that I want to wear amazing clothes and so on. Whatever floats your boat.

This exercise helps you to think longer term. Often, we can't think further than the weight. We fail to think about what our lives will actually be like, how different they'll be, how much better they'll be and all the things we'll be able to do that we can't, or don't do now. It's totally fine if you find this hard. This will change over time, and I recommend you come back and repeat this exercise in a few months as you learn more about how you feel when you love yourself. Your answers will be very different from when you don't.

ACTIVITY 14: SHARE YOUR SUCCESS

Sharing is caring, as some people say. Well, I say that sharing helps you get positive reinforcement for your great work. Sharing can give you the thumbs ups, the well done, and the OMG you're so awesomes - whatever stage of your journey you are on.

Sure, sharing on social media is not for everyone, but it works for many. Some use it as an accountability partner, others use it just to keep a record. Then there are those who use it to find friends, supporters, and cheerleaders. I used it to get inspired by other people on a similar journey, to learn new ideas, and to get involved in a community. I enjoy sharing my self-love and weight loss journey and I liked hearing about other people's successes too. Sharing has done a lot for me, and I think it can do a lot to boost your sense of achievement too.

1. If you're looking for a community of like-minded self-love and weight loss enthusiasts, I recommend posting on Instagram with all the relevant hashtags. Use the following hashtags for sharing your progress and for finding others on a similar journey:

#selflove
#iloveme
#loveyourself
#loveyourselfandloseweight
#consciouseating
#eatconsciously
#weightlossjourney

2. Follow me on Instagram

@loveyourselfandloseweight

Follow me because I would love to hear how it's going. I want to hear whether my self-love tips have worked for you, whether you enjoyed the book, what progress you're making. I want to hear all about your success!

3. Check out www.loveyourselfandloseweight.com for blog posts and the odd newsletter and to let me know how you're progressing on your journey.

4. Keep everyone else up to date with your success too. Sometimes it harder to talk to your friends and loved ones about weight loss than it is with random strangers on social media. Find a way to bring them into your journey with updates whenever you feel comfortable.

5. It's all very well telling other people about your success, but you also need to remind yourself of

everything you have achieved. Tell yourself when you're starting to feel it in the self-love department, tell yourself when you see the inches or pounds dropping off, tell yourself when you feel more confident, fabulous, and awesome.

6. Celebrate! It's important to celebrate you; to celebrate that you're loving yourself, to celebrate you're seeing results, all of it. Don't forget to celebrate by treating yourself at minor milestones.

7. Enjoy! Most of all, really most of all, enjoy this journey. Enjoy yourself. Enjoy every day.

Afterword

Thank you for reading my book. Thank you for keeping an open mind. Thank you for knowing deep down that self-love is the key to all of this.

I am excited that you're embarking on a self-love journey, and I'm keen to hear how it goes. And if there's one last thing that I'd like to let you know it's this:

I never thought I'd be able to help anyone else with self-love or weight loss. I never thought I'd write a self-help book, let alone a self-help book about self-love or weight loss. I never thought I'd post pictures of myself looking slim on Instagram or anywhere else for that matter. I never thought I'd lose 85 pounds and be a healthy weight. I never thought I'd love myself. And I never thought I'd ever, in a million years go for a run, wear a sleeveless top, or eat healthy food out of choice.

If I can totally change my life through learning to accept, then like, then love myself, then so can you.

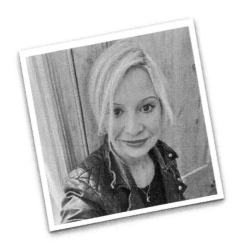

About the Author

Katie wrote her debut book Love Yourself & Lose Weight to share her experiences of successful and enjoyable weightloss. Having struggled with weight for many years, Katie found the secret was self love. This simple book about love aims to help people to love themselves, lose weight and be happy.

Katie is an author, speaker, artist, coach and entrepreneur. Having enjoyed a successful career as an award-winning innovator, Katie set up her own business to help people around the world to learn to love themselves, lose weight and find happiness.

Katie lives in Buckinghamshire, England with her husband Paul and daughter Lana.

Find out more about Katie at www.katielips.com and check out www.loveyourselfandloseweight.com for more self love and weightloss resources.

Get a free book!

As a thank you for buying Love Yourself & Lose Weight, I'd like to offer you a free book.

Seven Days to Self Love

Seven Days to Self Love is my free, no-nonsense guide to kickstarting a self love journey. Want to know how to go from feeling lack in the self love department to feeling head over heels in love with yourself in just seven days?

Seven Days to Self Love is yours for free if you head over to: www.loveyourselfandloseweight.com/7days

Get your free copy now!

A request...

Love Yourself & Lose Weight is my first book and I'd love to hear what you think. Did you enjoy reading it? Does my story resonate with you? Are you starting to love yourself and lose weight?

Please, please, please leave me a review on Amazon, or where ever you bought the book.

Please also check out my website at: www.loveyourselfandloseweight.com for more self love and weightloss resources, news about events, and more books coming soon.

Thank you!

Katie

xxxxx

Printed in Great Britain
by Amazon

79896385R00155